HOW TO GET A CELEB's BODY

ABOUT THE AUTHOR

Elise Lindsay has made her name as a top personal trainer, choreographer and fitness presenter. With over twenty years' experience in professional dance she is renowned within the fitness industry for her unique flair and teaching style. She won the prestigious title of Pure Energy Presenter in 2002 and in 2004 was named runner-up in the FITS Awards as Best British Newcomer. She has since gone from strength to strength and is now the celebrity's choice for all aspects of personal training.

For more information visit her website at www.eliselindsay.com

MICHAEL JOSEPH

Published by the Penguin Group
Penguin Books Ltd, 80 Strand, London WC2R 0RL, England
Penguin Group (USA) Inc., 375 Hudson Street, New York, New York 10014, USA
Penguin Group (Canada), 90 Eglinton Avenue East, Suite 700, Toronto, Ontario, Canada M4P 2Y3
(a division of Pearson Penguin Canada Inc.)
Penguin Ireland, 25 St Stephen's Green, Dublin 2, Ireland (a division of Penguin Books Ltd)
Penguin Group (Australia), 250 Camberwell Road,
Camberwell, Victoria 3124, Australia (a division of Pearson Australia Group Pty Ltd)
Penguin Books India Pvt Ltd, 11 Community Centre,
Panchsheel Park, New Delhi – 110 017, India
Penguin Group (NZ), 67 Apollo Drive, Rosedale, North Shore 0632, New Zealand
(a division of Pearson New Zealand Ltd)
Penguin Books (South Africa) (Pty) Ltd, 24 Sturdee Avenue,
Rosebank, Johannesburg 2196, South Africa

Penguin Books Ltd, Registered Offices: 80 Strand, London WC2R 0RL, England

www.penguin.com

First published in 2008

1

Text copyright © Elise Lindsay, 2008
Foreword copyright © Coleen McLoughlin, 2008
Photography copyright © Iain Philpott, 2008

The moral right of the author has been asserted

Designed by seagulls.net

Printed in Italy by Printer Trento S.r.l.

A CIP catalogue record for this book is available from the British Library

ISBN: 978-0-718-15337-3

Calorie counts taken from *The Calorie, Carb and Fat Bible 2007*, Weight Loss Resources, 2007

All sportswear provided by Nike

HOW TO GET A CELEB's BODY

Discover the secrets of the stars with your own personal trainer

ELISE LINDSAY

MICHAEL JOSEPH
an imprint of
PENGUIN BOOKS

With constant, fond and loving memories of my grandfather,
and heartfelt wishes for future strength and happiness for my grandmother.
Granddad, I hope I made you proud;
Grandma, I hope I continue to make you proud.

I'd like to dedicate this book to the wonderful inspiration of my life,
my best friend and role model, who I look up to and across to every single day:
Mum, you are my hero!

ACKNOWLEDGEMENTS

Firstly I'd like to thank my family and friends, especially my mum who is in the shadow of all my emotions. To Stacey, Jo and Ali, who from the start have been behind me and beside me, keeping the pages turning, through thick and thin … your words were always appreciated and your silences heard.

Thanks to Coleen for your constant efforts in training, putting up with my demands and laughing at my bad jokes!

Thanks to Kate my publisher, Chantal and, of course, Sarah, who has been on the phone endlessly taking care of every single detail. Thank you to Iain, the wonderful photographer who saw the person I am and to my agents for introducing the idea and forming a wonderful relationship with Penguin.

ve more

ould like to receive more information on Healthy
es, authors, special offers, events and giveaways,
email HealthyPenguin@uk.penguingroup.com

CONTENTS

PRAISE FOR ELISE LINDSAY

'Elise gave me back my life. Three years ago, youth left far behind, stiff and in pain, "I'd rather stay in than go out" – I showed all the signs of "the bad back". With sympathy, intelligence, humour, determination and enthusiasm – such enthusiasm! – Elise set about my transformation. The notion of "can't do" is foreign to her and so, mindfully and carefully, she took me on a journey which did, quite literally, give me back my life' *Alice McLure*

'Elise gave me a second life. A few years ago I feared I would have to give up my part-time work due to back pain and related migraines. My physiotherapist sent me to Elise and now I successfully manage a full-time job' *Isabel Díez*

'I think it would be no exaggeration to say that Elise has changed my life. She has incredible knowledge, experience, energy and enthusiasm and uses all of these to make sessions with her fun but still very productive. My posture has improved immensely, I am able to see the changes in my body shape and I look forward to continuing progress' *Jo Hookway*

'Elise is my flexible friend. Enthusiastic and always positive, for three years she has helped me to fight the physical ravages of middle age and a dodgy back. I leave my sessions with her both calmer and taller! I cannot recommend her highly enough' *Caroline Denby Hollis*

FOREWORD
BY COLEEN McLOUGHLIN

I first met Elise in 2005 when we were training for my fitness DVD, *Brand New Body Workout.* I had found it difficult in the past to stick to an exercise routine, but with Elise all that changed. She's the most energetic, enthusiastic and positive person I know – if anyone can make exercise fun and rewarding it's Elise. Her workouts have made a definite impact on the way I look and feel, and within just weeks of starting her programme I had loads more energy and could really see the difference in my figure. When I went on holiday that year I couldn't wait to try on my bikini – when you've worked that hard for something you feel really proud of the results!

It's not only my body shape that has changed while training with Elise, but my attitude too; she gave me loads of other tips and tricks on looking and feeling great that you'll find throughout this book. She covers everything, from your head to your toes and everything in between – it really is an all-over body workout! You'll learn about healthy eating, better posture, exercises tailored to suit you, and even how to look good in photos. The best tip I learnt was the 30% rule (read on to find out more!) – follow this and I'm sure you'll end up with a flatter, more toned stomach and improved posture so you will feel taller and slimmer too. I haven't looked back since working with Elise, and if you choose her as your personal trainer you will look and feel fantastic too.

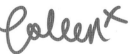

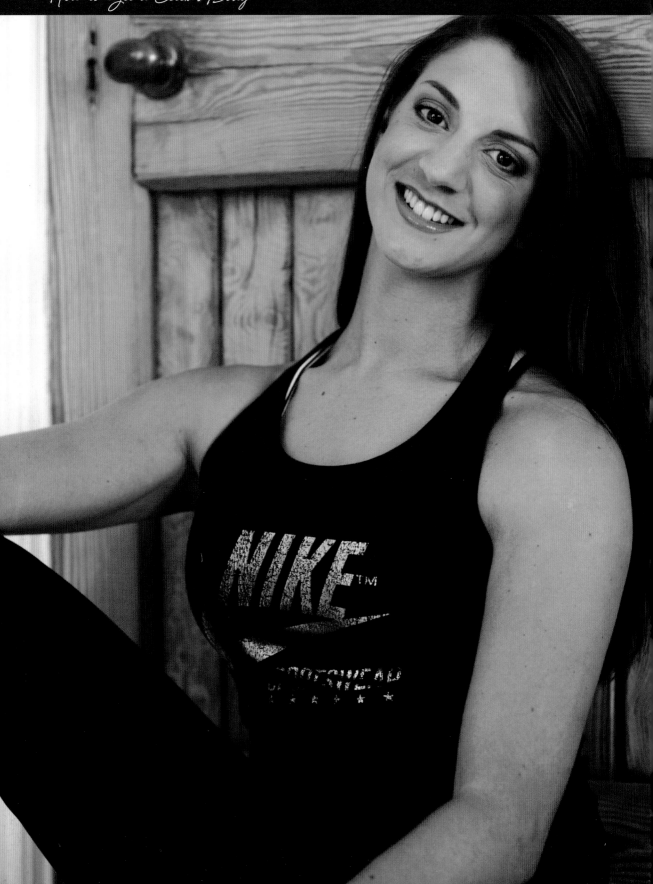

INTRODUCTION

a s I am sure most of you are aware, hundreds of diet books have been written and you may well be asking yourself what makes this one different. So I'll let you into the secret – the easiest and most effective way to look and feel fabulous is to add exercise to your life, and this book is designed so you can make small changes to your lifestyle that will guarantee a big difference in how you feel, look and are seen by others. In these pages I will become your personal body coach. I will give you a whole range of exercise plans to follow that will work on all areas of your body. In other words, I will be working on you inside and out (even muscles that you never knew existed!). Together we will take a look at your emotional and physical states and your eating patterns. There will be no difficult diet you have to follow for ever, but changes you will be able to make and maintain without a struggle. My aim is to offer you a realistic way of life, not to make you do something that seems like a punishment. You have taken the first step to a new you by opening the book; it's now time for us to get acquainted and move forward.

Let me introduce myself. I'm Elise, and I dedicate my time and energy to people. Working together I promise you will become my next success. Life is a gift; how we choose to live and enjoy it is up to each one of us. I was brought up to live life to the full and follow my dreams. This has led me to become very passionate about the things I do. As a young dancer I understood and appreciated the importance of technique, ability, goals and 'show time'. This has helped me immensely in my career; I have released several fitness DVDs, worked in television as a choreographer, presenter and dancer, and appeared at fitness and dance events at both national and international level. I have moved on from being a teacher to a trainer, then master trainer, and now find myself writing numerous articles for newspapers and magazines as a fitness expert.

I am credited with helping turn Coleen McLoughlin into one of the most glamorous-looking celebrities in the world. Photographs of her fantastic face and body have been flashed around the globe as interest in Coleen and her fiancé, football superstar Wayne Rooney, grows. Her new shape has transformed Coleen from shy schoolgirl to style icon, and I'm very proud to have led her through the personal fitness regime that has resulted in this transformation.

I first met Coleen in 2005 when I was asked to train her for her fitness DVD, *Brand New Body Workout*, which was released on Boxing Day that year. Following the DVD release we continued to train together and I can honestly say that Coleen is one of the best clients I have ever had. As with any client it was important at first to find out what her goals were. These goals then became my goals; achieving them became a joint effort and I became her dedicated fitness trainer/buddy and friend. I also gave Coleen nutrition and dietary advice so she could make speedier changes to her body shape and could feel the all-over benefits of good health and well-being.

Initially the rewards began to show in little ways – Coleen started seeing pictures of herself in the papers taken as she was leaving the gym, for example. The more we compared the before and after pictures, the more we could see the difference. Coleen's figure began to change, and she was delighted with the results. Her legs and bottom tightened up very quickly, she lost weight, although the real difference was in her increased muscle tone. Photographs of Coleen on the beach in Dubai really showed how far she had come – she looked fabulous. They also caused much speculation as to how she had got such a great new body.

This book will show you, step-by-step, how you can achieve the same results as Coleen and get the body you've always dreamed of – a body that will look every bit as good as a celebrity's. Not only will the book help you achieve your dreams, but it will provide a no-nonsense approach to getting and staying fit for life.

I am fully aware how hard it is to take the first steps on a new path, and I am also aware you may feel intimidated when going into a gym for the first time or taking on a personal trainer at home. Well, rest assured this guide will help you achieve a wonderful figure without slaving for hours in a gym. I have suggested a range of exercise programmes for you to try, from 10-minute energy workouts to more advanced and challenging timed circuits (an exercise programme that is fast and non-stop) working the entire body. Stress-beating breathing techniques and relaxation are also covered. All these different tools will help you make significant changes in your life.

Quick tips will help you make an instant improvement to your figure. How would you like to lose a couple of inches around your waist immediately so you can fit into your jeans without dieting? Impossible, you may think, but here's one example of how it can be done – many more tips like this are in the book.

- Imagine you have just taken a freshly washed pair of jeans out of the wardrobe and although you know they fit, they somehow seem a little small.
- Stop … relax. Lift your ribcage away from your hips, lengthen and grow – you may even have got a bit taller!
- Now you've found a waistline, imagine you have to fasten the button on your extra tight, just washed jeans.
- Breathe out to restrict tension elsewhere and then draw your navel in towards your spine, just to the point where you can still breathe easily, and keep it in.
- Go to a mirror and look at your reflection … instant shape change.

Your body will also be changed by focussing your mind on your goals. When mind and body work in harmony optimum results can be achieved more quickly, and they will last. Your mind has the ability to 'change' the body's natural pattern and re-programme it – in simple terms, give it an upgrade. Here's an example of what I mean:

- Stand up, join your hands together, arms outstretched in front of you (*Charlie's Angels*-style!).
- Rotate as far as you can and note the point that is directly in front of you. Hold the position for a few seconds.
- Return to the starting position, close your eyes and focus your thoughts on what is around you. Take a good 'look' around the room.
- Slowly rotate again, keeping your eyes closed. Remember what was in front of you before. Imagine going beyond this point. What would be in front of you now? See it clearly in your mind's eye.
- Return to your starting position, keeping your eyes closed.

- Keep focussing on your point beyond the original one, and then imagine going even further.
- Open your eyes and rotate again.

Well, what happened? Did you get further? The mental image should have led to an actual physical improvement. You made what seemed impossible ... possible! You see, this may not be so difficult after all! So far, you have lost a few centimetres from your waistline, without any dieting, and turned your body further than you thought you could without even considering your flexibility ... and this is only the introduction. *How to Get a Celeb's Body* isn't just about exercise techniques, it's a holistic guide to making changes in many aspects of your life, from diet, to fitness regime, to positive thinking. All of these will work together to bring out the best in you.

In Chapter One we'll look at the health benefits of staying fit and learn more about fitness myths and truths. Chapter Two will look at maintaining the body's balance with food by keeping a food diary and following a simple detox plan to kick-start your regime. In Chapter Three you'll learn how to build the body and in Four and Five you'll learn how to maintain that body for good. Chapter Six will look at just how easy it is to apply these techniques to your normal daily lifestyle. You will learn how to appreciate your body and increase your confidence, without it becoming a fixation.

This short guide is not just about becoming a fitter, healthier, happier person but about finding out who you really want to be. Take on the whole ride and enjoy the challenges and tasks you set yourself, the goal lines you have to cross and go beyond. This is a foundation upon which to build – it will allow you to gain structure and confidence that will stand you in good stead throughout your lifetime. Welcome to new ideas, beliefs and workouts to get you started on your own path to a healthier, happier you. Together, let us find that celebrity within you.

1
A NEW
WAY OF LIFE

Your journey begins with a new attitude! The only way you can achieve success is to see the changes you make becoming a way of life: this is a lifestyle, not a quick fix. Make gradual changes and remember that patience is a virtue. Initially this concept may be quite hard for some people to accept, especially if they have been lured into the traps of the commercial diet industry which promises instant results. But don't worry, you're not on your own – most people have tried the latest diet or bought an expensive product that claims to shed the pounds in a few days only to be let down in the long run.

There are many health benefits to be gained from being fit: you'll be less at risk from heart disease and other illnesses, less prone to PMS and you'll be feeling an inner and outer well-being every day. As you tone up and lose weight there will be less pressure on your joints, your skin will become clearer, your eyes will begin to shine and your hair will glow with health. You are also less likely to come down with colds and other bugs that attack weak immune systems. Coleen found that as she went through her training week by week she could really feel those health benefits. Her hair was sleeker and her skin looked amazing. She began to feel lighter and more confident. Being fit really does reap major health rewards.

Diets don't work because they offer a one-size-fits-all, rigid, eating plan which does not take into account the differences between individuals. If you are going to change your life you must take the following into consideration:

- your current eating pattern
- your current food choices
- your likes and dislikes
- your budget
- your exercise commitments
- your time availability

Don't be fooled by fancy marketing and miracle products. Why is the commercial diet industry one of the biggest and most profitable industries, when latest figures reveal that over 50 per cent of people in Britain are overweight and this figure is rising? Media hype and social pressure are the predominant reasons why so many people feel compelled to endure a painstaking diet. Fad diets are unlikely to prove successful in the long run and may even increase the risk of disease as many miss out vital vitamins and minerals. There are no miracle diets. Sorry!

And just in case you were unsure, there is also no diet that will make you lose weight from a particular part of your body. Think about it logically and it really doesn't make any sense at all. Unfortunately our society is rife with promises of quick fixes and easy methods for weight loss. It's a myth. The truth is that all you need is knowledge, a variety of tools and the right attitude.

The first step is to throw away your scales (or at least stop jumping on them several times a day!). Measuring body fat is undoubtedly the most effective way of monitoring body shape. In fact, find a pair of jeans that feel a bit tight, put them in the back of your wardrobe and leave them there. Try them on after six weeks. If they fit better then the diet's working – it's as simple as that. Weight measurement is an over-rated concept fuelled by media hysteria and modern-day nonsense about what makes the perfect body and thus the perfect life. It's rubbish! Thin doesn't equal happy. Start judging the quality of your life by how you feel, not by how you think you should look. In the long run this is the greatest gift you will ever give yourself. Negative self-image and low self-esteem can be precursors of obsession with weight. Take a good look inside

Measure who you are with positive thoughts and self-confidence, not pounds and inches!

> ## 'The Man Who Thinks He Can'
>
> Life's battles don't always go
> To the stronger or faster man.
> But sooner or later the man who wins
> Is the man who thinks he can.
>
> *Walter D. Wintle*

yourself and start to measure who you are with positive thoughts and self-confidence instead of pounds and inches!

Your first step on the road to a fulfilling lifestyle is to re-prioritize. A positive attitude, well-being and vitality must be at the top of your list. If you achieve this, a change in body shape for the better will be an inevitable by-product. Start today with a clean slate, banish those preconceived ideas and myths and just have one thought: 'I can do it.'

Goal-setting is key to achieving the results you want. How good does it feel when you are at work and you meet your targets, or when you have accomplished everything that you set out to do in a day? You feel proud of your efforts, and realize how much you can do when you put your mind to it. Goals can be made on a small scale, like going for a walk, or on a major scale, like fitting into that skinny pair of jeans you had hidden at the back of the wardrobe! Stepping stones of achievements provide a positive forward direction, and changes that occur gradually are easier to maintain.

Start by making a simple goal that you can achieve today and appreciate the feeling of completion – going to bed half an hour earlier, or swapping the afternoon cup of coffee for a herbal tea. Tomorrow, move on to something a little more challenging that you must complete by the end of the week, like fitting in a twenty-minute walk every day. Enjoying all the positive outcomes of achieving your goals will not only give you more confidence, it will ensure that other people notice the changes in your attitude and appearance as well.

Getting motivated starts here. Studies have shown that the decision to change a certain behaviour or lifestyle is made by weighing up the pros and cons, so that is exactly where we are going to begin. Write a list of all the pros and cons for reaching your goal. By reinforcing the pros and moving into action you will feel stronger and more motivated. Recognizing the cons will allow you to accept them and work out strategies for handling them effectively. For example, here is a typical list you could begin with:

PRO	CON
Feeling of achievement	Fear of failure
Intrinsic and extrinsic value (i.e. how you feel inside and what comments you get from others)	Other people being jealous of your success and achievements
Productivity within managed time	Hectic lifestyle
Having structure in life	Don't enjoy strict routine
Enjoying healthy food	Missing takeaways and luxury foods
Self-control	Feeling alone
Habit-forming	Too many existing bad habits
Long-term change	Wanting instant fix
Look and feel amazing	Feeling miserable at moment

The following research by two American psychologists explains a little about the behavioural changes you may go through on your new regime. Prochaska and DiClemente claimed that people who change successfully move through four stages:

- Pre-contemplation: in your mind the cons outweigh the pros, so you see no reason to change.
- Contemplation: the pros begin to outweigh the cons, so you are much more likely to take action.
- Action: you're feeling motivated and starting to get into a routine.
- Maintenance: you're focussed on staying at a level where you won't give in to temptation.

The key is to see the four stages as a cycle of events, so if you do slip up on your diet or exercise plan you should keep going. Concentrate on the positive change you decided to make until it becomes a way of life. If you feel yourself weakening, pick up your list of pros to remind yourself how much you have to gain from sticking to your new routine.

2
HEALTHY EATING, HAPPY YOU

great! So now you've decided to take a significant step towards a new you. What you put into your body really determines how you look, feel and ultimately how your body functions. You may have been eating the wrong things for many years. The only way to try to undo some of the damage you have done is to make a note of everything you consume, from regular meals to snacks and drinks – alcohol included! Once you have a clearer idea of your eating habits, you'll be ready to devise a diet and fitness plan that works specifically for you.

MANAGING YOUR RELATIONSHIP WITH FOOD – A FOOD DIARY

A food diary is an important tool with which you can carefully analyse your consumption of food and drink over a predetermined period of time to find out accurately the types, amount and quality of food you take on board and its benefit to you and/or the activity programme you are undertaking. It will give you some extra help in structuring your lifestyle. You should start recording your food and liquid intake as soon as you can, and make sure you include the amount of water you drink. You may wish to copy the sample daily grid over the page and use it to make weekly comparisons. Be truthful and record everything. The aim is not to make you feel bad, only to increase your awareness skills and allow you to look at your daily input. A food diary will help identify whether there are any emotional aspects that trigger or influence your eating behaviour. As you become more aware, it will also allow you the time to ask yourself if you are hungry, or if you are just trying to change the particular way you are feeling. If this is the case, try and do something else that will change this temporary feeling for the better. Simply filling out the diary will probably help you make positive changes. It's the oldest trick in the book – but it works!

It's up to you how long you keep the diary for; a week to a fortnight will allow you to see what sort of eating patterns you have, a month will be a good source of reference. When you are hungry and think it's time to eat, give yourself a hunger rating from the following list:

1 faint and weak
2 starving
3 quite hungry
4 hungry-ish
5 neutral

6 satisfied
7 full
8 stuffed
9 bursting and bloated
10 sick

DAY ......*Monday*......

MEAL	HUNGER RATING (OUT OF 10)	FOOD EATEN	AMOUNT	FULLNESS RATING (OUT OF 10)	THOUGHTS AND FEELINGS
Breakfast	3	Cereal and toast	150g and 2 pieces	6	Still a little bit peckish
Snack					
Lunch					
Snack					
Dinner					

Tips on Food Intolerance

Ever wondered if you are intolerant to certain foods? Many of us are without even realizing it. Intolerances come about when your body is unable to break down certain types of food or your stomach lining becomes hypersensitive to specific molecules in food which affects their ability to be assimilated properly. Allergies to food are generally a reaction of the immune system and are triggered by specific foods. Most commonly recognized allergies are triggered by smell, touch, fluid, inhalation or injection. Effects can be immediate and occasionally quite serious – a reaction to nuts and bee stings are probably the most obvious examples. If you think you may be allergic to a certain food you should see your GP for a correct diagnosis and further tests.

Feeling tired and bloated? This could be the result of a food sensitivity so it's time to crack down on your main offenders!

To find out if you have an intolerance, try recording the immediate and delayed effects on the body after food consumption, including your emotional state and energy levels. Take your resting pulse first thing in the morning (record for 15 seconds and times by four). It should be between 60–100 beats per minute. Then take it again immediately after eating. If your beats per minute have risen by over ten you may have a mild food sensitivity and should look out for any noticeable side effects. Keep a check when eating foods from a similar food group so you can eliminate anything that doesn't agree with you. Some food sensitivities are mild and temporary with symptoms such as gas, belching, bloating, fatigue, diarrhoea, constipation, skin rashes and mood swings.

Food sensitivity tests are becoming more easily available and provide guidance to finding healthy solutions within the common diet. The most usual sensitivities are to wheat and dairy products. Removing the offending food gives your body the opportunity to deal with the effects of the intolerance. When you reintroduce the food after six weeks or so, your 'clean' system should be able to cope with it.

TIME TO DETOX

Now you've learnt to manage your relationship with food, you're ready to kick-start your journey to the new you with a detox. Open those kitchen cupboards and have a good clear out. Get rid of all those things you know are really bad for you – anything high in fat, salt or sugar – the foods you know disagree with you and all those half-eaten jars of things that have been there for ages. Then stock up the cupboard with lots of healthy foods, and the fridge with fruit and vegetables.

After the detox, you can reintroduce foods back into your diet and see if any of them affect you negatively. If so, hey presto – maybe you should consider leaving that particular thing out of your general food intake. This is not just about losing weight either: by undergoing the detox you will find that, in general, the body works a lot more efficiently. By stripping down to find your body's natural balance you are creating the foundation blocks on which to build your body the way you want it.

Kick-start Your Detox

The liver and kidneys are the body's natural detoxers, as is the lymphatic system, but if you overload the body with toxins so that these organs can't cope, the toxins will never be completely removed from the body. So a detox allows the body's system to cleanse and repair itself from the effects of stress, bad foods and toxins that are taken in through food and drink and never fully released. Besides giving you a head start to achieving weight loss, if you detox you can expect to have better skin, nails and hair as well as more energy and better sleep. The body has to work constantly against everyday demands and fight the toxins we feed it, and as the pressures of modern life mean we tend to work more and look after our bodies less, in general we have lower energy levels than ever before and consequently more sickness.

If the body is finding it hard to keep pace, the performance of the kidneys and liver may suffer and, as a consequence, we simply slow down. The detox process stops the body being overloaded with toxins, provides it with a good selection of nutrients that promote cell renewal, cleanses the system while eliminating old toxins and gives you renewed strength and energy.

Detoxes usually spell misery so, if they are too hard to follow, after a few days you are likely just to give up and go back to your old habits. My detox is designed to clear out the system, yet takes into account that you also have a life and don't want to spend the next few weeks feeling miserable. I have made it fun and easy to do and you will start to really enjoy the way you are eating and the good you are doing to your body.

Make sure you *only* spend 14 to 21 days on this detox plan. It can be used to kick-start your regime or used any time you feel the need to 'clear the wardrobe'. Just follow the steps overleaf and you will feel like a new person in just a fortnight. Just a word about what you drink – make sure you have a minimum of a litre and a half of water per day.

Record your detox plan in your food diary, so you can see how your energy levels change as you adjust to the new diet. Many of my clients notice benefits of a detox very quickly. They start to feel less lethargic in the afternoons and have more energy for their training sessions. This also means it takes less time for their body shape to transform, which is an added benefit!

Detox my way, and feel like a new person in days!

Detox Plan

EAT ONLY	DRINK ONLY
fruit (only one banana every other day)	fresh fruit juice
vegetables (one portion of potatoes once every 2 to 3 days	herbal teas
i.e. a small baked potato or 3–4 small boiled potatoes)	milk – rice/soya/almond
salad	still mineral water
grains – millet, brown rice, rye, buckwheat, quinoa	
guacamole	
hummus	
lentils	
nuts (not caramelized or salted)	
oat/rice cakes	
porridge (with water or milk as listed, honey to sweeten)	
pulses	
Quorn	
seeds – pumpkin, sesame, sunflower, etc.	
soba noodles/wheat-free pasta	
sultanas/raisins	
wheat-free bread and crackers	

DO NOT EAT	DO NOT DRINK
dairy products	alcohol
eggs	fizzy drinks (including
fish	carbonated water)
meat	tea/coffee/any caffeine-based
ready meals	milk – cow's or goat's
sauces/dressings/mayonnaise	
sugar/sugar products: sweets, chocolate, cakes, biscuits, etc.	
white rice	
wheat bread	

Some Ideas for Detox Meals

- hot water with lemon and honey
- homemade muesli (for recipe, see page 31)
- tomatoes and mushrooms on rye bread (for recipe, see page 32)
- lentil or vegetable curry with brown rice
- fruit salad or mixed vegetable/fruit salads
- guacamole with Ryvita
- falafel (from health food shops)
- ratatouille
- stir-fry vegetables in wheat-free soya sauce
- jacket potatoes with tomatoes
- vegetable soups with wheat-free bread
- vegetable kebabs
- Quorn with brown rice and vegetables

Top Detox Tips

For maximum effect you may wish to follow some of the tips listed below. They will make your detox have maximum effect and make you feel good in both your body and mind while on and after the programme.

- Dry skin brush as often as possible using a small firm natural bristle brush available from most chemists. Dry brushing removes dead skin cells and aids circulation and lymph drainage. Gently brush a dry body, starting from the ankles and brushing upwards towards the heart. Brush the arms towards the chest. Avoid delicate areas and do not brush the face.
- Keep your body warm to help your circulation.
- Take a multivitamin for the duration of the detox.
- Sleep as long and as often as you can.
- Take a regular protein supplement mixed with water at least twice per day (minimum 60g).

There are many varieties of protein supplement available from health food shops – one of the best on the market comes in the form of a shake which is great after a training session, and quite filling. There are also bars available, but whatever you choose check the label, as some are designed to build muscle so can be calorific.

Spotting the Side Effects

Occasionally there can be some side effects when you are on a detox. Here's what they may be and how to alleviate them if they occur.

- **Headaches:** a possible result of reducing the caffeine content your body is used to. Tiger balm dabbed on the temples should relieve and soothe (see Star Supplements for extra help).

- **Increased urination:** this is your body eliminating the toxins. It holds onto water in an attempt to dilute offending food in the body. If the food has been removed, the result will be that you urinate more. And of course you will be drinking more water than normal. Sip your water rather than gulping it down. That way you take in less air which helps the body absorb the water more quickly.
- **Stomach problems:** as a result of the increase of fibre in your diet you may notice you are going to the toilet more, but if you are used to a large quantity of caffeine – thought to stimulate the bowels – the reverse may happen and you may become slightly constipated, in which case you should increase your fibre intake.
- **Cravings:** if you are craving a favourite food, this is usually the psychological effect of banning or restricting it. Try to stay positive and think of all the benefits your body is getting from the detox. Firstly see if you can take some exercise which will make you feel better and fill some time before your next meal. But you may get cravings because you are eating less and are still feeling hungry. It may be that your portions are too small, so slightly increase the amounts of porridge, rice and/or any food from the list that fills you up. Have some ready prepared snacks such as crudités. If, when you are peckish you don't fancy the snack options, chances are you are not truly hungry.

Star Supplements

Although what you eat will usually be the main source of nutrients, providing everything the body requires to function normally, during the detox process you may need some vitamin supplements and herbs to enhance your diet. There is a range of supplements to choose from and most are available from health food shops in liquid, pill, tea and powder form so ask for assistance to avoid confusion. If you want to add supplements to your diet I would suggest first taking a daily multivitamin, as this is a good source of everything then, if you wish to aid your detox further you could add no more than two other supplements. Seek further assistance if you are not sure which would benefit you most, but below are some suggestions:

- milk thistle – supports the liver and helps with initial headaches
- spirulina – purifies the blood
- Icelandic kelp – boosts metabolism
- multivitamin with iron
- chlorella – antioxidants A, C, E
- dandelion tea – helps reduce bloated feeling and fluid retention. Contains high levels of potassium.
- probiotic – aids digestion (you can include a probiotic by eating yoghurt)

HEALTHY EATING

Once you have finished the detox, you may slowly resume an ordinary healthy eating pattern but with care and attention. Reintroduce foods back into your diet one at a time and see how your body reacts – you may be surprised! If you have any food intolerances you will usually notice within 24 to 48 hours of reintroducing a particular food.

A balanced diet will give you bags of energy and glowing skin so don't hold back on the fruit and veg!

To live a healthy, energetic life you need to provide your body with the right foods, in the right portions and eat them at the right times. You need a balanced diet that supplies all the vitamins, minerals, protein, fat, fibre and carbohydrate you need. You should aim to eat at least five portions of fruit and vegetables a day (a portion is roughly a handful or cupful). These foods are known as nutrient-dense energy-light foods. This means they contain few calories yet hold an enormous supply of the vital nutrients we need for good health. Five a day is in fact a minimum requirement designed as an achievable goal for the public. The ideal consumption of fruit and vegetables is actually three to five portions of vegetables and two to four portions of fruit per day.

Carbohydrates are the main providers of energy. By eating a slow release carbohydrate like whole grains and rice the body's fuel lasts longer, and thus we don't feel the need to snack as much. This is because carbohydrates contain dietary bulk (fibre) which leaves us feeling full and is essential to the digestive system. You should have half a cupful or about 80 grams a day.

Healthy proteins are readily available, present in foods that many of us already eat as a standard part of our diet, such as animal proteins from meat and fish. But some have more health benefits than others – my advice would be to stick to white meat, such as chicken, and fish when following a healthy eating plan as these contain less fat and calories than red meats such as beef.

Fats should be present in our daily diet as they help nutrient absorption. Some fats, however, can be bad for your health, increasing the possibility of heart disease, high cholesterol levels and blood clots. Good fats are traditionally called monosaturated and polyunsaturated. These originate mainly from plant sources, for example, olive oil, oily fish rich in Omega 3 or nut oils. Bad fats are more commonly known as saturated or trans fats. These originate mainly from animal sources and tend to be solid at room temperature – think of the solidified fat from the traditional Sunday roast! Trans fats are often

> *Top tip*
>
> Try to minimize the amount of processed or ready prepared foods that you consume. Grill, don't fry, where possible, and replace vegetable oil with olive oil. Snack on nuts between meals instead of biscuits, buy the leanest meat available and trim visible fat away before cooking.

found in processed and commercially packaged food like microwave meals, biscuits or fast food French fries.

The following nutritional information will give you an idea of the essential foods that will keep you fit and healthy.

Vitamins

A: for healthy skin, night vision, protection against infection. Found in eggs, milk, oily fish, red, orange, yellow and dark green vegetables, sweet potatoes and fruit.

B6 and B12: help the body to make proteins and the nervous and immune systems and red blood cells function properly. Found in meat, chicken, fish, seafood, liver, whole grains, nuts, beans, peas and citrus fruits.

C: maintains the growth and repair of tissue and the health of cartilage, bones and teeth. Found in most fruit and vegetables.

D: helps the body absorb calcium for strong bones and teeth. Found in dairy products, some oily fish, egg yolks.

E: is an antioxidant and helps protect against free radicals which destroy cells and may contribute to heart disease and cancer. Found in vegetable oils, nuts, seeds, leafy green vegetables, wheat, oats, sardines and egg yolks.

K: helps blood clotting for repair to wounds. Found in leafy green vegetables, liver, pork, milk and dairy products.

Minerals

Calcium: for bones and teeth. Found in milk and dairy products, leafy green vegetables, canned fish and tofu.

Iron: important for our red blood cells. Women are commonly more deficient in iron than men due to losing blood through the menstrual cycle. Iron is better absorbed when eaten with foods rich in vitamin C. Found in meat, fish, poultry, soya beans, lentils, kidney beans, leafy green vegetables.

Antioxidants

Antioxidants are the nutrients in our food that can prevent and slow down the damage caused to our body from free radicals produced naturally when our body cells use oxygen. Antioxidants aid the immune system and therefore reduce the risk of infections.

Quick Immune Boosters

- Grapefruit has immune boosting anti-bacterial properties.
- Cranberries are great for helping cure urinary tract infections and have anti-fungal properties.
- Beetroot is an antioxidant with anti-inflammatory and detoxifying properties.
- Blueberries are rich in antioxidants.
- Broccoli is rich in antioxidants and iron.
- Garlic has anti-bacterial, anti-fungal and anti-viral properties.
- Ginger is great for circulation.

Sodium (salt): keeps a balance between the inside and outside of cells, but too much salt results in high blood pressure. There is no need to add salt to your diet as the body receives enough through natural foodstuffs. Salt reduction is often seen as a greater benefit. Avoid too much processed foods as these tend to have very high salt levels. Found in milk, fresh vegetables.

Fibre

You also need to include fibre in your diet. This is a type of carbohydrate commonly known as roughage which aids digestion and allows foods to pass through the digestive tract easily. Insoluble fibre moves waste quickly through the intestines and soluble fibre binds with bile acids and helps eliminate it. Found in dried peas, beans, lentils, chickpeas, kidney beans, vegetables, wholegrain cereals, oatmeal and brown rice.

Foods to Watch Out For!

Wheat: bread, pasta, beer, biscuits, desserts (containing wheat flour), etc. Too much refined wheat in your diet can have a negative effect on the blood and organs, and foods made with refined flour are particularly bad. However, don't worry about eating foods made from wholegrain wheat in moderation as it contains lots of fibre. If you want to reduce weight, reduce the amount of wheat-based foods you eat.

Dairy: milk, eggs, butter, cheese, etc. Cow's milk can be hard to digest and can sometimes cause allergic reactions due to the high fat content. However, remember it is a very good source of protein and calcium, so the key here is to use lower- or reduced-fat versions. Calcium can also be obtained from green leafy vegetables.

Refined sugars: processed foods of all sorts, biscuits, sweets, chocolate, cakes, fizzy drinks. Sugary foods are really addictive so the more you eat, the more you'll want – so do try and avoid them altogether. Too much sugar causes blood-sugar imbalances that can result in mood swings and although sugary foods can be a quick fix for immediate energy this hyperactive mood will soon change and you'll feel lethargic, depressed or anxious. Remember, sugar is incredibly addictive – the more you eat the more you want. You may also find it helpful to cut out fizzy drinks, including sparkling water. Many slimmers fill up on these types of drinks, but the gas they contain simply ends up in your stomach. Sugar replacements like sorbitol, maltitol or mannitol can also have a laxative effect and leave you with discomfort.

Not too Much!

If you know that you eat too much, here are a few tips to avoid temptation:

- Cut down your portion sizes (a portion is the amount you can hold in your hand, for grains about half a cup).
- Eat your food slowly and chew it well.
- If you can't live without hamburgers, avoid the fast food shops and buy a burger made of lean meat to grill at home.
- When eating out don't order super-sized meals.
- Share a starter with a friend.
- Don't eat from a family-sized bag of snacks. Pour some into a bowl to avoid overeating.
- Buy food packed in single portions when out shopping.
- If you don't enjoy food without sauces, cut down on the amount of sauce you would normally have.
- If you are used to seeing a big plate of food and portion sizing looks like a punishment change the portion sizes around so that the biggest portion is made up of vegetables and salad. Or put your food on a smaller plate!

Eat the Right Things at the Right Time

Another great technique to ensure you are not overeating or eating at times when you don't need to is simply to listen to your body's signals. Like cars the body is designed to work off fuel, so if it runs low or out of fuel the red light comes on and tells you it needs some more. We know that keeping the car regularly topped up with petrol is the best way to keep the engine ticking over smoothly rather than letting it run on empty, ready to shut down with a judder. When suddenly replenished in one go and filled to the brim, the car, though full, may seem heavier and sluggish. Likewise, to ensure our bodies tick over efficiently without any worries of slowing down we need to consult our food gauge.

Take another look at the chart on page 14 that rates your hunger. It's good to stay between zones 3 and 7 for optimum balance. If you wait until you are starving or feeling faint you may end up eating more than your body needs. Try to stop eating when you have reached 7 as anything you eat from here onwards will be unnecessary extra calories and will be stored in the body as fat. The more you try to listen to your body's natural signals the more you will learn about your eating habits.

Try to avoid eating when feeling emotional. This can distract the brain so it fails to register you are eating at all and therefore has no fullness signals to work from. Instead try and deal with the situation that is making you feel that way without resorting to food for comfort.

'Grazing' through the day is a beneficial way of keeping the body topped up with energy. If you are eating suitably sized portions at mealtimes but you still feel the need to eat snacks, there is a wide variety of fruit and vegetables you can snack on. Raw vegetables are great, you can eat most of the vegetables listed below raw, but some you may wish to cook in advance or simply save a few items from your main meal, put them aside and eat cold or reheat when required. You may wish stock up on any of the following and eat them, guilt-free, whenever you like. Just remember to eat when you feel a little hungry and stop when you are satisfied:

- apples
- asparagus
- bananas (but limit these to one every other day)
- beansprouts
- blackberries
- broccoli
- cabbage
- cauliflower

- celery
- cherries
- chicory
- courgettes
- cranberries
- cucumber
- French beans
- gherkins
- green beans
- lettuce
- mange tout
- mango
- melon
- nuts and seeds (but in small portions)
- peas fresh from the pod
- pears
- peppers
- plums
- radishes
- rocket
- satsumas or clementines
- spinach
- spring greens
- tomatoes

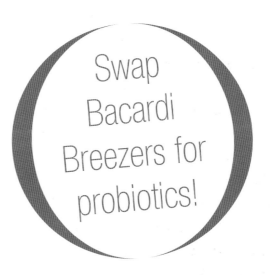

Swap Bacardi Breezers for probiotics!

Breakfast is undoubtedly one of the most important meals of the day. It kick-starts your day and your metabolism and gives you fuel to think and perform. If you don't eat this important meal you will find the body simply does not operate effectively; it's harder for it to find energy from stored carbohydrates, proteins and fats and therefore it makes it harder to lose weight. Your digestive tract may gradually weaken and this can affect the digestion of other meals. Even a small snack or a selection of fruit is better than skipping breakfast altogether.

Eating a good source of carbohydrates at breakfast and lunch is a great way of keeping energy levels up and hunger at bay. In the evening, eating proteins and vegetables and fruit which are easily digested is better for aiding rest. In simple terms your body does not need energy to rest – it needs to replenish. Providing the body with high-energy foods late at night will result in storage.

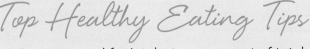

Top Healthy Eating Tips

- Decrease total fat intake to 30 per cent of total calories.
- Eat less animal protein.
- Eat more complex carbohydrates (starches).
- Eat less sugar.
- Eat more fruit and vegetables.
- Eat more fibre-rich foods (unrefined starches/ fruit and vegetables).
- Decrease salt intake.
- Drink more water.
- Moderate diuretic intake (caffeine and alcohol).

A FEW RECIPE SUGGESTIONS

It's often difficult to think of things to make so here are a few suggestions to start you off.

Breakfast Options

Hot Water With a Slice of Lemon (Serves 1)
Starts the digestive tract working and aids bowel movement.

Homemade Muesli
You can make up as much or as little of this as you like, and vary the quantities of the ingredients until it's how you like it.

For the basic dried mixture:
porridge oats
rye flakes
millet flakes
dried apple
dried papaya or mango
sunflower seeds
pumpkin seeds

Add fresh to taste:
raspberries or blueberries
pinch of cinnamon
rice milk
1 tsp of honey

Make up an airtight tub of the basic mixture by combining the dry ingredients.

To prepare, pour a small bowl of the muesli, add rice milk and a sprinkle of cinnamon, cover, and place in the fridge overnight. In the morning, add fresh berries and enjoy! If you forget to prepare it the night before, or you want something warm, you can pour over half and half rice milk and water, pop in the microwave and heat up before adding the fresh fruit.

Tomatoes and Mushrooms on Rye Bread *(Serves 1)*

2–3 tomatoes, diced

3–4 mushrooms, diced

olive oil

soy sauce

Worcestershire sauce

black pepper

1 slice rye bread

Edam (optional)

Stir-fry the tomatoes and mushrooms in a little olive oil (or place under the grill for a few minutes and then transfer to a pan). Once the tomatoes have softened and the mushrooms are cooked, season to taste with a little soy sauce, Worcestershire sauce and pepper. Serve on rye bread and grate a small amount of Edam on top.

Fruit Crumble *(Serves 1)*

Any combination of: apples, pears, papaya, pineapple, cherries, peach,
   plums, berries

1 heaped dessertspoonful probiotic low-fat yoghurt

1 wheat-free ginger biscuit

Cut the chosen fruits into small pieces, put in a bowl and add the yoghurt. Crumble the biscuit on top.

Smoked Salmon on Corn Thins *(Serves 1)*

2 small slices smoked salmon

2 teaspoons fat-free probiotic yoghurt

2 corn thins

Put one slice of salmon and a teaspoon of yoghurt on each corn thin and serve as a snack or a healthy breakfast.

Lunch Options

Vegetarian Chilli *(Serves 4)*

1 onion, chopped

1 clove garlic, finely chopped

2–3 carrots

red or yellow pepper

2 courgettes

vegetable oil

1 packet Quorn mince

large handful of tinned aduki beans

2 teaspoons mixed herbs

½ teaspoon chilli powder (or to taste)

1 tin chopped tomatoes

Stir-fry the onion, garlic and vegetables in a little oil until slightly softened. Add the Quorn, beans, herbs and chilli powder and stir. Cook for 2 minutes. Add the tomatoes and simmer for at least 10 minutes and up to 30 for a fuller flavour. Serve with salad.

Salmon and Steamed Vegetables *(Serves 1)*

handful broccoli, cut into florets

2 carrots, cut into chunks

handful green beans, chopped roughly

1 salmon steak

salt and black pepper

Steam the carrots and broccoli and after about 15 minutes add the beans and cook for a further 5 minutes. Grill the salmon for 5 to 8 minutes on each side and season to taste.

Spicy Vegetable Pot *(Serves up to 4)*

vegetable oil

1 onion, sliced

2 x 2cm pieces fresh ginger, sliced or grated

1 fresh chilli, deseeded and chopped

2 cloves garlic, chopped (optional)

1 yellow pepper, diced

2 courgettes, sliced

6 mushrooms, quartered

cumin, coriander to taste

1 jar passata

1 butternut squash, peeled and cubed

2 carrots, diced

salt and black pepper

1 tin mixed beans (optional)

Heat the oil in a large saucepan and stir fry the onion, ginger, chilli, garlic, pepper, courgette and mushrooms. Add the spices. Add the passata, the butternut squash and the carrots. Simmer slowly for 50 minutes. Season. In the last 10 minutes you may add a tin of mixed beans as a spicy bean pot alternative!

Coriander and Lime Quorn Stir Fry *(Serves 2)*

350g Quorn

juice of a lime

1 teaspoon ground coriander

vegetable oil

1 onion, finely sliced

1 red pepper, sliced

handful beansprouts

small tin water chestnuts

¼ Chinese leaf or cabbage, finely shredded

1 carrot, cut into thin strips

Marinade the Quorn in the lime juice and coriander for at least 2 hours. Stir fry the onion until softened and golden. Add the remaining vegetables and any remaining marinade and cook for 5 to 10 minutes. Grill the Quorn for 5 minutes and serve on top of the vegetables.

Bean and Vegetable Casserole *(Serves 4)*

1 onion, chopped

head of broccoli, broken into pieces

2–3 carrots, sliced

tin kidney beans

tin chickpeas

tin tomatoes

2 vegetable stock cubes

1 fresh chilli, deseeded and sliced

2 teaspoons curry powder

1 x 2 cm piece ginger, grated

1–2 cloves garlic, crushed

Pre-heat the oven to 190°C/gas mark 5. Put all ingredients into an oven-proof dish. Add some water until the vegetables are just covered. Cover with foil and put in the oven for 30 to 45 minutes.

Dinner Options

Have the soup as a first course, followed by the chicken salad below. Remember you can make twice as much soup if you want, and can then save or freeze any leftovers.

Carrot, Celery and Coriander Soup *(Serves 1)*

> 1 stick celery, finely chopped
> 2 carrots, finely chopped
> 1 vegetable stock cube
> handful of fresh coriander, chopped
> black pepper

Put the celery and carrots in a saucepan and just cover with water. Add the stock cube. Bring to the boil and simmer for 10 minutes, stir in most of the coriander, reserving a little for a garnish, then simmer for a further 15 minutes. Allow to cool slightly then blend the mixture until it reaches desired consistency. Garnish with the remaining coriander and season with pepper to taste.

Chicken Salad *(Serves 1)*

> few spears asparagus, cooked
> 1 chicken breast
> handful salad leaves
> handful sundried tomatoes

few baby tomatoes, halved

50g feta cheese (optional)

small handful pine nuts

small handful pumpkin or sesame seeds

balsamic vinegar

Bring some water to the boil in a saucepan and add the asparagus. Simmer for 5 minutes. Drain.

Meanwhile, steam or grill the chicken breast (one per person), chop and put in a serving bowl with the salad leaves. Include flavoursome leaves such as rocket and herbs to make the dish as tasty as possible. Add the sundried tomatoes, baby tomatoes, asparagus and a few cubes of feta cheese if you wish. Add the pine nuts and seeds. Dress with balsamic vinegar.

Vegetable Stir-Fry and Brown Rice *(Serves 1)*

¼ cup brown rice

olive oil

1 onion, finely chopped

1 clove garlic, chopped

2 cm piece fresh ginger, finely chopped

selection of vegetables: choose from green beans, broccoli florets, mush-
  rooms, sugar snap peas, baby sweetcorn, spring onions, water chestnuts,
  bamboo shoots, beansprouts

1–2 tablespoons honey

handful of fresh coriander, chopped

dash of balsamic vinegar

salt and black pepper

For the salad:

handful fresh baby spinach

Cook the rice as per the instructions on the packet. Season to taste.

Meanwhile put a little olive oil in a pan and stir-fry the onion till softened then add the garlic, ginger and vegetables and cook for about 10 minutes. Once the vegetables have softened, add the honey, coriander, balsamic vinegar and seasoning.

Serve with a salad of spinach and the rice.

Dessert Options

Summer Fruit Surprise *(Serves 1)*

> *small bowl frozen summer fruits*
>
> *1 tablespoon fat-free probiotic yoghurt*

Defrost the fruit for 5 to 10 minutes (it's more like a sorbet if they are still part frozen, but defrost according to your preference!) and top with the yoghurt.

Cheese and Biscuits *(Serves 1)*

If you enjoy cheese and biscuits as a dessert try a couple of wheat-free ginger biscuits each topped with 1 teaspoon low-fat cottage cheese.

BBQ Banana *(Serves 1)*

> *1 banana*
>
> *cinnamon or nutmeg*
>
> *2 teaspoons fat-free probiotic yoghurt*

Place a banana in its skin straight on the barbecue and cook it for about 10 minutes or until the skin is black. For the indoor version … grill the banana until black, turning when required. Or peel a banana, wrap it in foil, and bake in the oven at 190°C/gas mark 5 for 10 minutes or until soft. Sprinkle with cinnamon or nutmeg and serve with the yoghurt.

Fruit Salad (*Serves 2*)
>   *apple*
>   *grapes*
>   *orange*
>   *pear*
>   *pineapple*
>   *plum*
>   *fresh orange juice*

Slice and deseed some or all of the above fruits, and cover with the orange juice. You could also try some exotic fruits in season.

FEELING JUICY?

How about making a fresh juice that contains some healthy vitamins and nutrients? Have juice for breakfast or any time during the day but preferably not with meals because the sugar in the fruit may ferment in the gut making it harder for the body to digest the food. For added energy, to help your immune system, to detox and for a great skin try:

- **Pineapple, apple, carrot and celery:** contains folic acid, vitamin C, calcium, magnesium, manganese, phosphorus, beta-carotene, sodium and sulphur.
- **Apple and blueberry:** contains beta-carotene, biotin, folic acid, vitamins B1, B2, B6, C and E, calcium, chromium, magnesium and sodium.
- **Apple, carrot and ginger:** contains vitamin C, calcium, magnesium, phosphorus, potassium, sodium, sulphur and beta-carotene.

Experiment with different fruits to come up with a variety of juices. Include vegetables and make a smoothie. Write down the recipes of your favourites. You may wish to try a rich smoothie first thing in the morning if you are training or have one during the day as a pick-me-up and stomach filler. Smoothies will keep fresh in the fridge for a couple of days. Try blending:

- mango, pineapple and passion fruit
- strawberries and banana
- banana, pineapple and orange
- apple, pear and strawberries
- melon, kiwi and pear
- mixed berries, apple and banana
- blackberries, raspberries and blueberries

For a thicker version add 3 to 4 tablespoons of bio yoghurt to the fruit. Experiment with seasonal fruits to ensure you get a great helping of vitamins and minerals essential to your new well-being plan.

Tips for Reducing Calories

- Choose foods labelled low fat (containing 3g fat or less per serving) or fat-free products which only contain 0.5g of fat, or less, per serving.
- Swap foods labelled 'enriched' for labels saying 'fortified'. Enriched products can lose nutrients while being processed whereas fortified products contain their original nutrients plus other vitamins and minerals.
- Swap family-size portions for snack-sized.
- Choose wholegrain bread, pasta and rice which contain more fibre and vitamin B.

Cooking Tip

Think about how you cook your food. Making a simple swap can also save you calories.
For example, here are the different calorie contents of an egg cooked in various ways:

- boiled: 88
- scrambled with milk: 148
- Scotch: 301
- omelette, plain: 115
- fried in oil: 107
- poached: 89
- omelette, cheese: 240
- 100g quiche with cheese and tomato: 274

Crack Down on Calories

Here's how to work out how many calories you need a day:

- At rest, the body uses 25 calories per kilogram of body weight. This is the basic metabolic rate (BMR).
- BMR for a 60 kilo individual is 60 x 25 = 1500 calories per day. This is the amount of calories you need to simply exist without doing any kind of activity.
- For different levels of activity we must add on the following percentages of a person's BMR:

  Sedentary lifestyle + 20 per cent

  Moderate activity levels + 50 per cent

  Very active lifestyle + 100 per cent (this only really applies to athletes)
- So if our 60 kilo person was moderately active we would add 50 per cent of their basic 1500 calories to their total:

  1500 x 1.5 = 2250 calories

If you are concerned that your current diet it too high in calories, try out some of the simple food swaps on the next page.

SWAP THIS	CALORIES	FOR THIS	CALORIES
homemade chips 200g	546	medium jacket potato	210
naan bread	336	2 chapattis	222
egg fried rice 250g	520	boiled rice 250g	348
2 large sausages	232	chicken breast	215
crisps 35g	186	pretzels 25g	99
milk 1 pint full fat	317	milk 1 pint skimmed	161
jam doughnut	252	hot cross bun	202
Cheddar cheese 30g	123	Edam cheese 30g	99
Greek-style yoghurt	180	low fat yoghurt	80
cheese sauce for pasta	197	tomato sauce for pasta	58
croissant	180	2 crumpets	160
white bread per slice	93	wholemeal bread per slice	74
cream cracker	31	wholemeal crispbread	17
potatoes roast 300g	447	potatoes boiled 300g	216
Caesar salad	374	plain salad no dressing	151
deluxe turkey sandwich with bacon and cheese	482	ham and turkey salad sandwich, no mayo	290
quarter pounder beef burger	386	quarter pounder veggie burger	240
pasta (50g) with pesto sauce	454	pasta (50g) with tomato sauce	271
1 serving creamy Caesar Italian dressing	68	2 tablespoon low calorie Italian dressing	4
1 can potato salad	274	medium jacket potato with 1 tablespoon light sour cream	239
minced beef 100g	239	minced turkey breast 100g	161
full fat Cheddar 100g	409	reduced fat Cheddar 100g	255

You can find the calorie content on most food labels. This will allow you to keep track of your consumption and not buy or eat things that will exceed the recommended daily intake. My only concern when looking at calorie content is that certain foods may appear high in calories but may be very good sources of vitamins or nutrients, for example, avocados, nuts and seeds. This does not mean you have to cut down on foods that may be an important part of your diet. You can make significant calorie reductions by swapping certain foods for others. Here is a short list of foods you may eat often, and an alternative which will reduce your calorie intake immediately. Here's a calorie guide to help you when choosing what meat to buy and how to cook it.

MEAT	PORTION SIZE	CALORIES PER PORTION
grilled back bacon	50g	152
roast beef	100g	136
roast lamb	100g	217
grilled lamb chops	100g	231
grilled pork chops	100g	240
roast duck	100g	423
roast goose	100g	319
roast turkey	100g	171
chargrilled chicken breast	100g	197

Healthier Takeaways and Eating Out

Takeaways are often very high in calories, and so are some dishes in restaurants. So you should try to restrict the amount you have. For example, a doner kebab and salad contains 300 calories, a ¼ pounder with cheese has 471 calories and a ¼ pounder with fries and coleslaw is a massive 658 calories! If you can't resist, there are some guidelines overleaf to calorie content and some alternatives so you don't have to choose the very high calorie dishes.

CHINESE

Fewest calories: boiled/steamed rice, vegetables, chicken, seafood

Most calories: fried rice, battered/deep fried, seaweed, prawn crackers

TYPICAL DISH	CALORIES	ALTERNATIVE	CALORIES
beef with green peppers and black bean sauce	380	beef in oyster sauce	340
chicken chop suey	425	chicken in lemon sauce	300
crispy duck, 4 pancakes	800	chicken and pineapple	310
prawn balls in batter (10) with sweet and sour sauce	1200	sweet and sour chicken	480
pancake roll	240	spare rib	140
prawn cracker	100	prawn toast	70
egg fried rice 100g	208	brown rice 100g	123

Fried rice has a very high calorific content so try this alternative: cook a portion of brown rice (half a cupful), then spray a little olive oil into a pan and stir-fry some chopped spring onions, frozen peas, finely chopped ginger and chopped garlic. Add a dash of soy sauce and some Chinese five-spice powder. Add the rice to the pan, stir and serve. Or, try this healthier alternative to beef in oyster sauce, which saves about 100 calories:

Chicken in Oyster Sauce (Serves 1)

> *vegetable oil*
> *1 onion, sliced*
> *1 garlic clove, finely chopped*
> *1 red chilli, de-seeded and chopped*

1 chicken fillet, sliced

1 red pepper, finely sliced

small handful broccoli florets

small handful mange tout

2 teaspoons soy sauce

3–4 tablespoons oyster sauce

Heat the oil in a frying pan and sauté the onions till soft, add the garlic and chilli and stir, then add the chicken and brown. Add the vegetables and cook for a further 10 minutes. Add the sauces, cook for a further 2 minutes and serve.

INDIAN

Fewest calories: pulses, chicken, jalfrezi, balti, tandori, madras, dupiaza, boiled rice, salad, seafood.

Most calories: fatty meats, fried dishes, pasanda, korma, masala, fried rice.

TYPICAL DISH	CALORIES	ALTERNATIVE	CALORIES
chicken korma	870	tandoori chicken	300
lamb bhuna	680	vegetable biryani	550
chicken masala	431	chicken tikka	396
chicken curry	700	vegetable curry	350
lamb rogan josh	403	vegetable balti	294
chicken dhansak	720	aloo saag	500
beef kheema	780	beef madras	540
onion bhaji	190	poppadom	65

To save a huge amount of calories, try replacing meat with Quorn.

Quorn Curry *(Serves 2)*

    vegetable oil
    1 onion, sliced
    350g Quorn
    1 clove garlic, finely chopped
    1 red chilli, de-seeded and chopped
    4 mushrooms, quartered
    1 red pepper, sliced
    2 tomatoes, diced
    1 teaspoon cumin
    1 teaspoon coriander
    pinch turmeric

Heat the oil in a frying pan and add onion and cook till softened. Add the Quorn, garlic and chilli. Then add the rest of the vegetables and the spices. Simmer for about 15 minutes. Serve with boiled brown rice.

Spicy Vegetable Wraps *(Serves 1)*

    vegetable oil
    1 clove garlic, finely chopped
    1 red chilli, de-seeded and chopped
    1 tin chickpeas, drained
    handful spinach leaves, washed, drained and chopped
    1 tin chopped tomatoes
    1 teaspoon Worcestershire sauce
    handful fresh coriander, chopped
    sweet potato, cubed
    1–2 plain chapattis
    fat-free Greek-style yoghurt

Put a little oil in a frying pan and stir-fry the garlic and chilli for a few seconds. Add the chickpeas, spinach, tomatoes and Worcestershire sauce and stir till the mixture bubbles. Add the coriander. Cook the sweet potato in boiling water for 10 to 15 minutes until tender. Sprinkle the chapattis with water and grill for 30 seconds on each side. To assemble the wraps, put some of the sauce on the centre of a chapatti, add 2 teaspoons of yoghurt and fold over. Serve with the steamed sweet potato.

ITALIAN

Fewest calories: vegetables, ham, tuna, chicken, prawns, tomato-based sauces

Most calories: pizza, pepperoni (on pizza), creamy sauces, garlic bread with cheese

TYPICAL DISH	CALORIES	ALTERNATIVE	CALORIES
garlic bread (4 pieces)	400	bruschetta	220
tiramisu	440	ice cream	140
lasagne	650	cannelloni	500
spaghetti Bolognese	720	spaghetti marinara	690
pizza	750	chicken risotto	550
spaghetti carbonara	1020	spaghetti Napoletana	630

A lot of pasta dishes have creamy sauces which are high in calories and pasta is, of course, made from wheat. Try an Italian feel with less wheat with my Garlic Prawns and Wild Mushroom Risotto recipes on the following page.

Garlic Prawns (*Serves 1*)

　　olive oil

　　8 cloves garlic, finely chopped

　　small packet peeled prawns

　　1 red chilli, de-seeded and chopped

　　50 ml white wine

　　salt and pepper

Heat the vegetable oil in a frying pan and add 4 cloves of garlic. Cook till softened. Add the prawns and chilli, and cook till the prawns change colour. Add the wine and season. Stir till the wine bubbles and serve immediately. You can have this as a starter or as a main course if you add rice as a side dish.

Wild Mushroom Risotto (*Serves 1*)

　　1 vegetable stock cube

　　half cupful Arborio rice

　　handful of mushrooms

　　1 clove garlic, finely chopped

　　handful fresh coriander, chopped

　　chilli powder to taste

Dissolve the stock cube in about 500 ml of boiling water. Put the rice into a pan and add enough water to cover. Simmer and stir until the rice has absorbed the liquid. Add a little more water, and the rest of the ingredients. Keep stirring and adding water until the rice has softened, absorbed all the liquid and is cooked (this takes about 20 minutes). Serve with a salad.

MEXICAN

TYPICAL DISH	CALORIES	ALTERNATIVE	CALORIES
beef chimichanga	765	chicken chimichanga	675
chilli con carne	800	chicken enchiladas	615
350g well-done sirloin steak with fries	860	beef enchilada	700
chicken fajitas	1035	vegetable fajitas	810
beef fajitas	1300	beef burritos	695

Mexican food can be high in calories and fat due to the creamy side sauces
– avoid them if you can. Try making these fajitas at home:

Fajitas (Serves 1)

    vegetable oil
    selection of vegetables or a chicken breast, cut into chunks
    fajita seasoning
    2 healthy option tortillas
    2 tablespoons low-fat probiotic yoghurt

    for the salsa
    200g tomatoes, skinned and chopped finely
    2 green chillies, deseeded and chopped
    1 small onion, finely chopped
    1 clove garlic, crushed
    1 teaspoon cumin
    Tabasco and salt and pepper to taste

Heat the oil in a frying pan and add either the vegetables or chicken and
stir-fry. Add the seasoning.

To make the salsa, mix all the ingredients and put in the refrigerator for at least an hour.

Assemble the fajitas: fill with the tortillas with vegetables, or chicken, top with yoghurt and some salsa. Serve with a salad and a low-calorie dressing. Try drizzling the salad with balsamic vinegar or make a honey and mustard mix and pour over to taste.

BRITISH

Typical calorie content in pub food

TYPICAL DISH	CALORIES	ALTERNATIVE	CALORIES
225g well-done rump steak with chips	525	pork and apple casserole	360
roast beef with trimmings	540	shepherd's pie	400
sausage and mash	585	fish pie	450
toad in the hole	640	Lancashire hotpot	400
beef stew with dumplings	770	beef casserole	490

A simple stew can be accompanied by boiled new potatoes, parsnips, steamed vegetables or rice – try this recipe:

Vegetable Stew (Serves 1)

> *1 leek, chopped*
> *1 small onion, chopped*
> *1 courgette, sliced*
> *2 carrots, cut in sticks*
> *a small handful of peas*
> *2–3 mushrooms, sliced*

vegetable stock cube

spices

salt and pepper

Preheat the oven to 180°C/gas mark 4.

Put all the vegetables in a casserole dish and pour over enough boiling water to cover. Add the stock cube, spices and seasoning, cover and place in the oven for an hour.

Suggestions for Eating Out

When you eat out it is very easy to have more calories than you intended. Simply having the side order of bread and butter, the chips or a sauce that is full of cream will pile on way more calories than if you had eaten at home. Don't be afraid to ask if the chef can adapt a dish to suit your needs – after all, it's what all the celebs do and little changes will make a big difference!

General

- Ask that a sauce be served separately so you can choose how much to have (this goes for salad dressings too).
- Ask for extra vegetables instead of potatoes.
- Ask how the meat or fish is cooked and see if you can have it steamed or grilled rather than fried.
- Choose lean meats or fish to reduce the fat content.

Italian

- Opt for tomato-based sauces rather than cream-based ones.
- Choose thin-crust pizza rather than thick to reduce the wheat content.
- Avoid pepperoni – this is quite a fatty meat.
- Avoid dishes overloaded with cheese.

Chinese

- Choose boiled rather than fried rice.
- Order dishes containing more vegetables – stir-fry dishes are a good option.

Indian

- Order plain boiled rice.
- Avoid naan. If you want bread choose chapattis.
- Choose tikka and tandoori dishes as they are cooked on a skillet without fat.

European

- Grilled, steamed, boiled and roasted dishes are generally the best option.

Mexican

- Without the sauces, most Mexican dishes are fairly low in calories. Choose grilled, boiled, roasted or steamed options where possible.
- Beware of all the dips: ask for them to come as a side serving or see if there are any low-fat options.
- Avoid too much cheese.

Top Food Tips

- If you want a sugar fix or an energy boost – hold off on the chocolate and cereal bars and reach for the fruit, dried or fresh, which will give you a natural sugar lift.
- Shop when you are full, not when you are hungry. Write a list so you can stick to your regime and avoid temptations even if they are on offer!
- Cut down on portion sizes gradually – it is not a punishment, just a slight change will make a big difference over time.
- Add different spices to foods like chicken, fish and rice.

- Try steaming vegetables instead of boiling: it only takes 15 minutes for most vegetables to cook and helps keep all the essential vitamins and minerals.
- Prepare two meals at once to cut down on the time you spend in the kitchen. Preparing a meal in advance means it only has to be warmed up when you get in, giving you a slot to work out in or some essential 'you' time.
- Make healthy, simple soups and stews – they are a fantastic standby and very quick to do.
- Record how long you actually sit down and put your feet up for. Instead of those biscuit breaks make sure you are active and save your resting for the pamper time when it's in your schedule.
- For dessert treats try a baked banana in its skin (cook in the oven for 20 minutes), open and serve with low-fat bio yoghurt and a drizzle of honey. Defrost frozen summer fruits and serve with low-fat bio yoghurt.
- Clear all the cupboards of anything that may allow you to give in to temptation.
- Get rid of the deep-fat fryer.
- Replace meat with Quorn which is high in protein and low in fat.
- Eat slowly so you can tell when you've had enough.
- Watch your liquid intake; energy drinks such as Lucozade and milky drinks like lattes are high in calories.
- If you're going on a night out, eat sufficiently before you leave to avoid the takeaway temptation later on in the evening.
- If you're a mum DO NOT eat the children's leftovers.
- Don't fall into the trap of eating ready-made convenience foods, you will be piling on calories! Stock up on tinned pulses, lentils, brown rice and tomatoes – healthy store-cupboard food that is quick and easy to cook.
- Plan your snacks, so whenever you get the mid-afternoon munchies you'll have something already prepared.

Drink

How much alcohol do you consume in a week? The recommended amount is 21 units for men and 14 units for women. Work out roughly how many units of alcohol you consume per week – a pint of beer or cider amounts to two units, a small glass of wine, or a measure of spirits is one unit. Find the drink you prefer from the list below and work out your calorie intake.

DRINK	CALORIES
pint of beer	182
can lager (440ml)	189
glass white wine (120ml)	87
glass champagne (120ml)	89
pint Guinness	170
measure vodka (25ml)	56
measure gin (25ml)	56
measure medium sherry (50ml)	58
measure Baileys (50ml)	175

Leave the bar behind and shape up those thighs on the dance floor!

If you want to reward yourself by having a drink, make sure you have an extra training session to compensate for the extra calorie intake or try to reduce your calorie intake for that day.

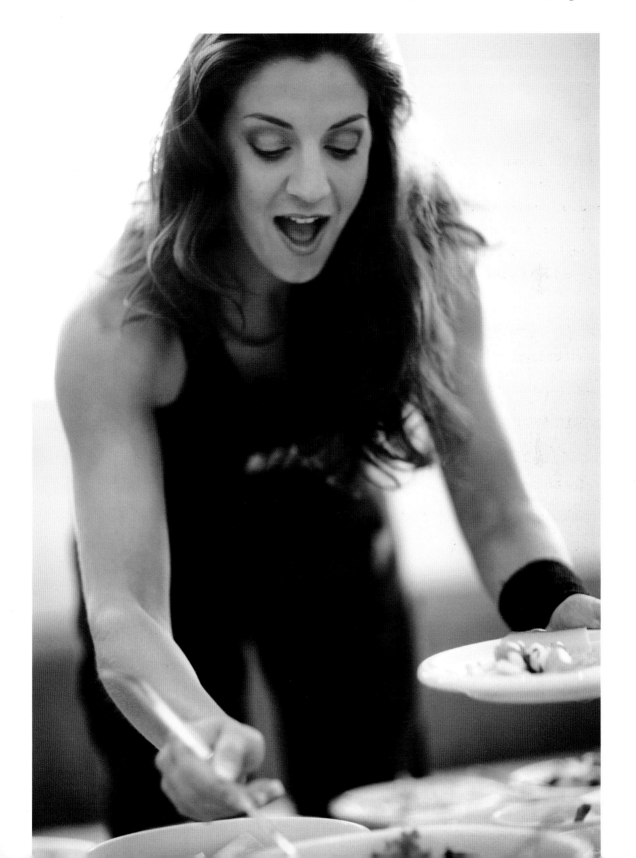

3
BECOME
SOMEBODY

So, now you've learnt how what you put into your body makes all the difference, it's time to start building that body. Different types of exercise produce different effects on the body. During cardiovascular activity you increase your heart rate and burn calories more efficiently. Weight training will tone your muscles, reduce body fat, and help you have a long and healthy life by reducing your blood pressure and bad cholesterol levels and reducing the chance of you getting osteoporosis. Core exercises are also a crucial component of fitness, and are often not performed enough. The core muscles (abdominal, back and bottom muscles) are responsible for maintaining stability in the body. The core is where all movement begins and it is only with a strong core that the rest of the body can experience maximum benefit from other types of exercise.

Getting up and active not only makes you feel good but burns calories – the best of both worlds!

You can start an exercise routine immediately. Simply getting up and active will burn more calories than sitting still and letting your body function with minimal effort. You should aim to increase your activity levels three to five times per week. You can choose to vary your level of effort from moderate to intense and this will determine how often the activity needs to be repeated. If you prefer to do a light to moderate workout there is no reason why you can't repeat similar activities on a regular basis or every day. If your workout is more intense your body may need a little longer to recover and therefore may need more variation. The workout section in Chapter Four (see pages 72–191) gives different levels to choose from, allowing you to increase the intensity of your workout as your strength and fitness levels improve. If you begin training while on the detox programme you may find your energy levels are a little lower than normal and as a result the workouts appear harder. Stick to a level that enables you to work well but which does not push you to the limit. While you are in the 'clear out' – the weakest phase – it is important that your workouts have a positive effect and make you feel good. The endorphins released through exercise should combat stress and enhance your mental health and well-being. Endorphins are the chemicals that give us the feel-good factor which is why, no matter how bad we feel sometimes about making the effort to get up and do something and no matter how difficult activities may appear to be, the feeling you get afterwards will be worth it. This is why exercise is recommended by doctors for people who may be stressed or depressed, for the uplift in mood it provides.

PREPARING FOR EXERCISE

Equipment

There are no essential requirements when it comes to exercise other than yourself, your workout programme, some space and some water. As you progress with your workout challenges you may wish to invest in some weights for increasing and decreasing your resistance. In the workout section on pages 72–191, you will be using resistance for some exercises. You do not have to go out and buy equipment immediately: you can save money by creating your own weights at home. A large bottle of water, for example, holding about a litre, will give you a weight of about a kilo. To have a selection of weights all you need to do is take empty bottles, socks or tins and fill them with different substances such as water (for light), sugar (for medium) or pebbles (for heavy). Make sure you have a pair of each weight.

A couple of dynabands will be useful – these are stretchy bands, often made of rubber, that come in various colours representing different resistances. You can perform many exercises with the bands and they take up no storage space at all, so you can use them anywhere – at work or on holiday.

A workout mat with a supported area or a yoga mat with a non slip surface is a great investment, but a towel will do just as well in the beginning.

Clothing

Wear what you feel comfortable in. A reputable make of sports bra with breathable fabric is a good investment for the times when you'll be working up a sweat. It's also a good excuse to go shopping as it's important for you to feel great in the clothes you wear for fitness.

For aerobic and conditioning activity, the basics are:

- sports bra
- trainers
- comfortable clothes

Invest in a pair of trainers that will support you during your workout sessions. It is important to realize that the different styles available on the market support different areas of the foot for specific activities. You may want to seek advice to find a good trainer that suits your foot and the type of activity you'll be doing. Get a general cross trainer to suit all your exercise needs and look later for a specific shoe if you find a preferred type of training. For example: while I wear running shoes for running, I prefer an aerobic boot for aerobics classes and dance as I turn and pivot more and need ankle support. You will find good advice in most shops or go to www.stepnpump.com for a wide selection of suitable footwear.

When you put on your favourite outfit, how do you feel? Why does it make you feel so great? Is it the shape, fabric, colour or cut that flatters you? Looking good also makes you feel good, so there are a few tips overleaf to help you find a workout outfit that makes you feel good before you have even begun!

Top Tips on How to Flatter your Figure While Training!

- Make your bottom and stomach appear flatter by wearing darker colours and slightly higher-waisted trousers.
- Use bright colours to accent your good areas and try gathered or detailed tops to smooth out any bumps or tight-fitting areas.
- Make your legs seem longer and more slender by wearing dark-coloured leggings. A boot-cut also makes the legs look longer as it balances the ankles in relation to the hips.
- Make your hips look smaller by wearing dark-coloured hipster trousers to give a lower waistline. Combine the trousers with a brighter-coloured top that matches the colour on the waistband. If you have a flat stomach do not be afraid to show it.
- Give yourself curves by layering tops to create form. For an athletic figure try cut-away necklines.
- Reduce curves by accenting the length of the legs: wear trousers with a vertical line down the leg. For tops, experiment with interesting neck lines and slight sleeves.
- Don't wear underwear that is too small; you are far better buying a bigger-sized pair of pants so you flatter your shape with a smooth line as opposed to having an unsightly dug-in knicker line because you have squeezed yourself into something too small because of the size on the label.
- Invest in a sports bra that fits you well and will give you the support you need. There's nothing more distracting (or uncomfortable) than wearing the wrong bra when you're out for a run!

Save Some Cash!

Exercising at home is a great money-saver – not only do you save yourself time and petrol money going to and from the gym, you will be saving yourself a fortune in gym membership. You could put aside your would be gym membership fee and save it for a big reward like a holiday!

Here are a few extra things you can do away from the gym to increase your energy output:

- Going out with friends – maybe even clubbing – watch your alcohol consumption and, at a certain time, stop and move on to something like soda and lime. Dance more instead of drinking.
- Arrange to do something as a group or with a friend like walking, swimming or even horse riding.
- Go roller skating or ice skating – more fun than you'd think!
- If you know you are going out, up your training – push yourself a little harder for a little longer!
- Go for a walk before dinner and vary your speed as an extra challenge.
- Leave the car at home and cycle instead.
- Take the stairs at work rather than using the lift.
- Do your daily jobs a little faster than normal (time yourself and log each activity – you can try and beat this each time!).
- Do some gardening.
- Play outside with the children.
- Take the dog for a walk.
- Wash the car rather than taking it to the car wash.
- Hide all remotes so each time you change channel you have to get up.
- Perform mild exercise in front of your favourite TV programme.

GETTING STARTED

To start you off, take a picture of your body. Then measure your waist, hips, thighs and arms and record the information. Write down how you feel now and what your energy levels are. Put the photo at the front of your training diary as a reference to the point at which you started – it will help you maintain your motivation. Record what you do every day and the times you do it – taking the children to school, going to work, eating lunch, washing up and so on.

When planning your exercise programme you need to dedicate a time slot to it. This way, it will be fixed in your schedule and become part of your daily routine. If your schedule is pretty hectic, look realistically at what things can be moved, shortened or changed so that you can fit your exercise time in.

Setting Targets and Reaching Goals

Goal setting is a simple yet often misused motivational technique which can provide some structure and a focus for your training programme. One of the most important things about setting a fitness goal is planning to reach that desired target. How many times have you decided to set about improving your body only to go flat out in the gym in the first two weeks and throw in the towel by the third, because you have pushed yourself too far and you don't have a plan? With that in mind I'm going to tell you how to plan effectively. Here are two well-known acronyms which are designed to help you achieve your goals and keep you on track. The first is SMART or SMARTER:

S goals must be **Specific**
M training targets should be **Measurable**
A goals should be **Achievable**
R goals must be **Realistic**
T training targets should be **Time-based**
E goals should be challenging and **Exciting**
R goals should be **Recorded**

So, for example your goal could be:

S *I want to lose 12 kilos and fit into my red dress for my friend's wedding.*

M *I will record my measurements and weight loss weekly to monitor that I am on target.*

A *yes, it's achievable based on losing a kilo a week.*

R *yes, this is realistic.*

T *4 months.*

And the basic principles of fitness training are summed up in the acronym FITT:

Frequency – how often
Intensity – how hard
Time – how long
Type – of training (strength, endurance, etc.)

Here's how you can use this acronym:

F *I'm going to train three times a week at home and go outdoors for a long cardiovascular workout. I will also incorporate some aerobic activity every day.*

I *I will work at beginner's level.*

T *a 45-minute training session and 30 minutes of aerobic activity every day.*

T *two general toning plus one circuit, walking and running programme.*

What Are Your Goals?

The first step is to identify what you want to look and feel like. What do you want? Are you looking to tone up, lose weight or improve your posture? How would you feel if you achieved this change? What difference would it make to every aspect of your life?

Once the process has begun, your brain, often unconsciously, will already have started to work out the procedure which makes reaching your goal a whole lot easier. Start to put together a comparison between where you are now and where you want to be. See it as a positive and realistic vision. Break your goal down into lots of mini goals that will eventually lead to your ultimate target. Sometimes a single goal becomes an evaluation of your entire worth, so don't place too much emphasis on the final result. You might miss out on the now! Celebrate every step and every little goal achieved. Write five self-praising statements every day.

Celebrate every step of your journey to fitness – appreciating the small achievements is the key to your success

Make a written contract for each of your goals as suggested opposite. It's a helpful tool in times of stress or weak motivation. Use it to remind yourself why you started this programme of change in the first place. Fully commit to your goal. Give it positive energy every day and results will be yours.

You will normally start to see some benefits over a four to six week period. Setting yourself a time frame is very useful. For example, a friend's wedding in ten weeks' time or a holiday in three months'. Believe me, having a goal will really keep you motivated – you'll be thinking how good you'll look on that beach or in that slinky dress.

When goals are set then reached it often drives people on to bigger and better things. For example, I have had clients who have never exercised before whose fitness levels have improved so much that they have run charity marathons. Other people have gone on to train to become personal trainers or instructors. In general, if you exercise you will simply look much better and stand out from the crowd.

Sometimes goals aren't reached because of time. It's important to factor in a realistic time frame, otherwise you may be disappointed when you don't achieve them.

Date	01.01.08
Description of goal	Tone up and improve general fitness.
Target completion date	1.06.08
Evaluation date	7.01.08. Re-assess 30.01.08. Weekly measurements and weight; monthly evaluation to confirm goal is still achievable and make amendments if necessary.
What will it feel like when I get there?	Sense of achievement, empowerment, happier, in control.
What do I need to do to achieve this goal?	Stay focussed and dedicated; follow my plan, work hard, manage my time effectively.
Plan of action from now until my evaluation date	Apply FITT, keep training and food diaries.

Achievability

Make sure your goal is achievable within the constraints of your existing lifestyle. Writing down what you want to achieve will help your commitment no end; it will represent a contract with yourself and will make working out part of your new lifestyle. If you are a size 20 as you begin, it's almost impossible that you'll be a size 10 by the end of an eight-week programme. You have to be realistic about your goals; remember you are not after a quick fix but are aiming for long-term fitness and health benefits. You wouldn't suddenly decide to become a runner and then enter a marathon the following week. By trying quick fixes you could be damaging your long-term goals. Giving yourself a time frame in which you expect to achieve these long- and short-term goals will allow you to look forward to some of the rewards you will gain when you've achieved them.

> Be realistic about your goals; remember you are aiming for long-term fitness and health benefits

Throughout this book there are exercises which you can vary to come up with a programme which is right for you. Ideally, you should do activities which increase your heart rate every day, and this can be achieved just by replacing a car journey to work with a cycle ride or by simply increasing the pace at which you walk to and from your destination. A good friend of mine once said 'Do you know what the first rule of dynamics is? Input always equals output.' We frequently hear phrases like 'What goes in must come out.' Well, I hate to be the bearer of bad news but our bodies are designed to take input and use some of it for output and store the rest of it up for later on. It's how much we store that we need to keep an eye on.

COACHING YOUR MIND

Believe in yourself. If you believe, you can achieve. Banish those negative thoughts! Popular culture tries to make us believe that unrealistic body shapes are the only way to achieve success and happiness. It is difficult to avoid the depressing effect this media-imposed idea of perfection has. We are not born with the instinct to self loathe – we learn it! Try out the following techniques and you'll soon see a difference in the way you think and feel about yourself:

Beat the Inner Critic

Write down all the things you *can't* do. It does not matter how big this list becomes. Take a final look at the list (maybe some of the things are still real, maybe some of them are beginning to look a little silly). Next, destroy the list – you may wish to burn or bury it. Let your 'I can'ts' rest in peace and begin living the life of 'I can'.

Outweigh the Inner Critic

Set aside some quiet time to think about what you have done recently. Do you begin to praise or criticize yourself? Try to praise your recent actions and diminish the 'would have', 'could have', 'should have' thoughts. Turn up the volume of your positive voice and weaken the negativity until it has gone.

Don't think that losing weight and improving your shape is going to be the hardest task you have ever had to do, it's easier than you think. The only thing you really have to lose is body fat, low energy and low self-esteem – now that sounds like a very good deal!

FIRST STEPS TOWARDS YOUR WORKOUT

To begin with, it's best to work on a general all-over body programme, to wake the whole body up but keep it balanced. It also allows you to recognise your current strengths and feel how your body operates. Take one of the basic primary fitness tests outlined on page 76. Record the results and use them as a point of comparison at a later date when the test is repeated. You'll be surprised at how quickly your fitness levels improve once you start exercising on a regular basis.

Once the body has started to develop some general strength and you can determine how often your workouts are going to take place it may be of greater benefit to target certain areas of the body and make them work harder, rather than allow these muscles a recovery day while another area becomes your prime focus. Using this method, muscle tones more quickly, but you have to be committed to your training timetable to ensure your body remains proportioned.

It is also worth experimenting with the time slots you train in and record them in your training diary (see page 82). You may notice performance and energy levels differ through your workouts depending upon the time of day. Make your workouts manageable within your timeframe but also be aware that your performance levels may vary.

Don't worry if you a feel a little sore the day after your workout. This is known as DOMS – delayed onset of muscular soreness, it will only last a couple of days. If it does last longer than this or you have swollen joints you have pushed yourself too hard. Remember, this will all get easier; it may take 21 days before things start to feel more comfortable in your new life plan but just keep going and aim to improve.

Top Tips for Personal Power

Here are some cherished golden rules – call them, if you will, my ten commandments.

1 Believe in yourself and expect to succeed. Allow your confidence to grow.

2 Learn from past experience but don't dwell on it, continue to find ways in which to move forward.

3 Congratulate yourself for the things you have achieved, no matter how small.

4 Be confident that the things you can do will always outweigh the things you can't.

5 When you are feeling happy it's time to train! It will make you associate a good feeling with working out. Whenever it gets hard, laugh it off; always try to have fun during your workout.

6 Ban the ban. Never ban something completely, this will result in constant torment and can often result in breaking the ban.

7 Never let anyone tell you that you cannot do something you set out to do, chances are the real reason they say this is because they can't do it themselves.

8 Don't expect miracles in your first few sessions and don't go reaching for the scales. Take your time.

9 Don't be afraid to fail: treat each minor failure as a learning curve for the future.

10 Never lose faith or step backwards, a sideways step for some time out is OK but always focus on the best way to move forward.

I want you to take these rules on board, write them down, keep them nearby and refer to them daily as a constant reminder.

REWARDS

Think about something you like doing or have always fancied doing; maybe the things you would love to do never happen due to lack of time, other commitments or priorities. Make a list of them, then cut the list into strips, put them in a box and allow yourself a surprise reward by drawing one out when you hit a target or achieve a goal.

Repeating the following mantra will also help you to focus on the progress you have made: I will try and try again until I master my successes – I know I will succeed as I have just taken my first steps.

KEEP A JOURNAL

Keep a journal to remind you of all your feelings. When things seem bad and you write them down, they often don't seem as bad anymore. When things feel great you have something to look back on and can reflect on that good feeling. It may also help you remember the actions you took. Similar situations and feelings can occur and you will have a greater sense of control by knowing how to move forward. Write down how you feel when you reach a goal. Look back on it often to remind yourself of that great feeling.

Tip for Success

If you have given something up, replace it with something else. For example, replace a cigarette break with a glass of juice; replace staying in and comfort eating with a walk, going to see friends or preparing a healthy snack.

REAL-LIFE SCENARIO

Exercise makes you happy – FACT!

After breaking my foot over the Christmas holidays, my training had become non-existent and I was trying to build myself back up, but felt weaker than ever before. But I was determined to get there.

I went running for the first time since my foot had been taken out of plaster ... I left the house in a pretty miserable frame of mind, having woken up tired and with no energy. I had grunted to my boyfriend that I was going running (and truth be told it was only due to a football kick-off and the thought of a 90-minute testosterone blast that pushed me to leave right then!). I put on his MP3 player and ran ... not only did I clear my head and solve a few problems that had been bugging me but, as I began listening to the upbeat track I was no longer short of breath or thinking about the weakness in my foot. I was in my zone, smirking to the delights of the drums and occasionally punching the air with a fist or a finger in a heat of disco heaven! My pace increased and decreased to the music and I know I had a better 'pushed' run than I would have experienced with silence and my thoughts alone. My music was my trainer, my support and my motivation. I felt lifted and exhilarated while pushing myself harder and harder. It was almost like the finale of *Chariots of Fire* as I hit the home straight. No sooner had I realized my run had been far more energetic than I had planned did I also realize my mood had switched! What was earlier a sluggish, grunting, lethargic girlfriend who could barely utter the words 'How are you today?' had become a girlfriend wanting to wrap her arms around the man in her life, voice her love for him and then get dressed in something fantastic! It's amazing how a bit of cardiovascular exercise can change your mood and possibly the direction of your day!

4
THE WORKOUT SELECTION

here's where we get started on the practical! This is it – time to go!

I'm going to introduce you to different types of training to give you a choice of what sort of exercise you can do. Remember this should be fun! You should enjoy the exercise as well as making an improvement to yourself. Don't be overwhelmed by all the different workouts; you are only going to do one to begin with and get really familiar with it before introducing another. The reason there are so many is that I know you will progress and need to challenge yourself – even though you may not think so right now. Your body will get stronger, your stamina will increase and, as you notice changes, I guarantee you will want to push yourself more.

If a workout doesn't feel right for you, adapt it or move on to another. What may work for one individual may not suit someone else. For example, one of my clients did not enjoy swimming but knew it had great benefits. I advised her to take up skipping instead, which she did. She even laughed out loud as she did it. Her skipping workouts moved her forward and as her fitness levels increased and she felt more confident in attempting more challenges she began to include a short swim in her routine. Her increased fitness and self-confidence shifted her negative feelings about a particular form of exercise to a positive experience of it. You have to enjoy your workouts – whatever they include – otherwise you won't stick with them.

I'm going to outline briefly some different forms of exercise . . . let's call it the 'here comes the science' part! Don't be afraid of the terminology or logistics, it's a point of reference and a way of increasing your knowledge.

TYPES OF EXERCISE

Aerobic Exercise

Aerobic exercise is an activity performed over an extended period of time which gets the large muscle groups working at a regular pace, makes you breathe harder and increases your heart rate. Aerobic exercise uses more calories than other activity and will make your heart stronger and more efficient. Some examples of aerobic activity include:

- brisk walking
- aerobics workouts
- bicycling
- swimming
- jogging
- running
- skipping
- roller skating
- tennis/squash
- using cardiovascular equipment (treadmill, cross trainer, rowing machine, exercise bike)

The factors affecting aerobic fitness are frequency – how often you perform aerobic activity; duration – the length of time you spend doing them; and intensity – the percentage of your maximum heart rate at which you work (see pages 79–80). Most experts believe you should spend 20 to 60 minutes on cardiovascular activity three to five times a week.

Conditioning/Strength Training

Conditioning means simply that – exercise that will keep you at your best. Strength training will increase the body's power and stamina which leads to toned muscles and a leaner appearance. So it is important that your training schedule includes exercises to build strength and to tone and condition the body. As with cardiovascular activity, strength training will improve the body's fitness levels as well as having other great benefits like increasing bone density, reducing body fat and making you more resilient to injuries. The aim of strength training is to increase the ability of the muscles used to exert or resist a weight or force. In other words, by putting muscles under pressure they adapt and become stronger. Many women fear that by lifting heavy weights they will bulk up and so avoid increasing effort levels. Women generally do not have enough testosterone to make bulky muscle and therefore increasing the level of effort will only benefit and complement the body's natural shape.

Core Training

It is essential to train the core muscles (the area between the navel and the spine – it's the powerhouse of the body that holds everything together) in every single session! If the core doesn't have strength the rest of the body subsides and has no clear way of development. The core is the foundation where all movement begins. Get this bit right from the start and not only will it prevent injury it will make other exercises easier. Movement starts from a strong core ensuring a safer workout and better overall end result.

Pilates

Pilates is a slower, more delicate type of exercise. This is not to say that it is the easiest form of exercise to tackle. It requires fine tuning, concentration and patience.

Using a steady breathing technique, exercises are designed to work the mind and body (tuning the mind to the muscle). By putting the body in challenging positions you promote the use of deep core muscles and back stabilizers. Stretching, mobility, balance and awareness are key factors in Pilates, and combinations of these are used in this form of body-shape training and correction methods.

FIND YOUR STARTING LEVEL

Throughout your training programme, it's important to monitor your fitness so you can see the progress you are making and find the right level of workout for you. The following exercises are not designed to determine how fit you are, they are just a selection of basic exercises that will allow you to see your starting point and measure your progress. They are only based on three elements, but you may choose to add or change these to suit you, for example, if you find running 1.5 miles quite difficult, start by walking briskly.

- Run 1.5 miles – how long did it take?
- One minute of press-ups – how many did you do?
- One minute of sit-ups – how many did you do?

Your results are only a guide to your overall fitness and are measurable only against yourself. Record the results and then do the same routine every month, at roughly the same time of day for a more accurate comparison, and record your progress so you can add it to your list of achievements.

WHAT'S YOUR BODY SHAPE?

I've given you exercises and workouts that will target specific areas of the body as well as workouts for all-over improvement (see pages 112–21). If you are new to fitness a great way of getting started is to work the whole body and feel the immediate benefits of training. As you progress and want to tailor your programme further, you may find the following body-shape information useful so you can determine your natural shape and work out how to start improving it.

Although genetics determine body shape, it can change with growth and development. You cannot change your fundamental body shape but you can make the most of what Mother Nature has given you by following a good diet and exercise programme.

There are three basic body shapes: endomorph, ectomorph and meso-morph. No one is 100 per cent one of these; we are a mixture of body-shape characteristics although one type is usually dominant.

- **Endomorphs** generally have a round build with big bones, large trunk and thighs and are prone to carry larger percentages of body fat. Shoulders may be narrower than the hips. Face shape is round.
- **Mesomorphs** generally have a muscular build, broad shoulders, narrow waist, naturally large muscles and fast metabolism due to the amount of lean muscle they have. Weight may be carried more in the upper body which will be compact or stocky.
- **Ectomorphs** generally have a light build, narrow waist, hips and shoulders. The ectomorph also has a low body fat percentage. An ectomorph has a linear appearance and an ultra-fast metabolism resulting in a slim appearance even when eating well. Ectomorphs may lack shape due to their low muscle weight. Lean muscle weight is what gives us that shapely figure.

The workouts which follow have sets (how many times you repeat the exercise) and reps (how many repetitions). There are intensity options to choose from as you progress. To help personalize your plan based on your body shape, use the following as a guide to the weight, level and speed at which you should train.

- **Endomorph:** fat loss is your main target so it is important that you are as active as possible. Regular cardiovascular training is essential and strength training should also be undertaken to help reduce fat and increase muscle tone. Exercise frequently and use moderate weights (2–4 kilos). You should aim to start the workouts at Level 1 (beginners), increasing to Levels 2 and 3. Rest periods between sets of exercises may be up to a minute when first starting out but as you progress gradually reduce this to 30 seconds. You should include a circuit session (see pages 168–77) as soon as you have mastered the basics! Try to eat smaller meals more frequently rather than large meals with long intervals in-between. And watch your intake of food – fats and sugars should be minimal or eliminated from your diet altogether.

- **Mesomorphs:** tend to have a naturally fit body and strength training can be performed with moderate weights (2–4 kilos) at a moderate pace. Vary your workouts between all levels and types of exercise. Rest periods between sets can also vary: when using lighter weights (1–2 kilos) reduce rest time to between 30 and 60 seconds and with heavier weights (5–10kg) increase it to between 60 and 90 seconds. Muscle can be gained fairly quickly so when you are happy with their size you can train to maintain. Vary your fitness activities and don't overdo it.

- **Ectomorphs:** gaining weight by increasing muscle is your main goal. You should aim to work between Levels 1 and 2. When working at Level 1 with maximum weights (5–10 kilos), the rest period between sets can increase to 3 minutes if needed or to the point when you feel recovered. (Avoid being distracted in your rest time; remember you still have work to do!) When working at Level 2 reduce the rest time to between 60 and 90 seconds, but still use it to recover properly. As you will be lifting heavier weights you may find it useful to invest in some dumb bells. Eat more food to increase your calorie intake but make sure it is good food and not junk. Keep aerobic activity minimal and don't train too often or for too long.

Tips to Help You Create Your Own Workout

If, over time, you have successfully used all the workouts, you may wish to select some of the exercises and put them together in a different order. This can have a positive effect on your training progress and you won't have to learn any more exercises. If you fancy having a go at re-moulding your workouts you may wish to consider the following tips:

- Start off with a basic workout on which you can build by increasing time or intensity.
- Don't get complacent with an activity or routine – the body simply adapts, making certain targets harder to reach.
- Notice your energy levels – are they higher in the morning or the evening? Train at the time you have maximum energy.
- Don't be too adventurous, keep SMART. Your workout programme can be from 30 to 90 minutes, but don't get carried away. Listen to your body and adjust to suit its needs.

HEART RATE

You should exercise at a level that raises your heart rate to your target zone. This is called intensity of effort. Your target heart-rate zone is 50 to 75 per cent of your maximum heart rate. To work out your maximum heart rate take your age in years away from 220 and then calculate 50 to 75 per cent of that number. The table on page 80 gives you a guide. To find your resting heart rate simply take your pulse for one minute.

Age	Average Maximum Heart Rate 100 per cent	Target Heart Rate Zone 50–75 per cent
20–30	195	98–146 bpm (beats per minute)
31–40	185	93–138 bpm
41–50	175	88–131 bpm
51–60	165	83–123 bpm
61+	155	78–116 bpm

Here's a little test you can do to see if you are working within your heart-rate zone. Count your pulse beats mid exercise for 15 seconds then multiply by 4 to get the beats per minute. If the result is faster than your zone you are working too hard and if it's lower this indicates you can push yourself a little more. When starting out you should always aim to work to the lower end – 50 per cent – to allow for improvement. As you get in better shape you can push yourself a little more to reach the higher end of the scale. Always try to work at a gradual, comfortable pace.

RATE OF PERCEIVED EXERTION

Another way you can monitor how hard you are working is called the rate of perceived exertion (RPE). This method is a lot easier than the heart-rate method, although less accurate, and is a nice way to stay in tune with your body and recognize challenges throughout your programmes. Perceived exertion is assessed by using a 1–10 scale to evaluate a combination of sensory feelings from your muscles and joints as well as your heart and breathing rates. You can therefore use the RPE scale at any time to gauge exercise intensity and monitor a comfortable workout.

1   rest
2   extremely low effort
3   low effort
4   very comfortable but noticeably working
5   comfortable but working
6   slightly uncomfortable but breathing regular
7   uncomfortable – can talk but must stop talking to catch breath
8   high effort, cannot talk
9   approaching extreme effort, difficult to breathe
10   extreme effort, cannot continue

Before you begin your exercise programme note your current breathing rate. It will probably be rated at one, then as your heart rate increases when you begin a cardiovascular activity to warm up, you may find you get a little short of breath. How hard are you working, or how much effort are you now putting in? The rating should have increased. As you continue and push yourself harder, once the body is warm, the scale should increase again. If the figure is still pretty low or only reaching 6, it's time to pick up the pace and increase your intensity (effort) level. If it has increased to 9 or 10 decrease the intensity of the activity slightly. You should never be able to hold a full conversation while you are working in your desired training zone, but you should also never be either speechless, exhausted or feeling faint. Over time you may notice that your recovery rate increases and it takes less time for your breathing to return to normal.

Use the following training diary or your food diary to record your activities
and emotions through the day. I've filled some things in as an example.

Training Diary

Date	Programme / time spent	Daily activity	Total time spent	Emotions
30.06.07	General 45 mins	Walking 30 mins Gardening 40 mins	1 hour 55 min	Feeling great/loads of energy
01.07.07	Circuit 50 mins	Jog 15 mins Cycling 20 mins	1 hour 25 min	Circuit tough, tired but pleased with run – may try run on day without circuit
03.07.07	Pilates 30 mins	Walking 30 mins Skipping 10 mins	1 hour 10 min	Definitely felt my muscles working and I enjoyed the skipping!
05.07.07	Conditioning 45 mins	Jog 15 mins Cycling 30 mins	1 hour 30 min	This combination worked well for me – not too tiring
06.07.07	Aerobics 30 mins	Walking 1 hour	1 hour 30 min	Walking good way to cool down after aerobics – feeling energised
07.07.07	Pilates 30 mins	Skipping 10 mins Walking 30 mins	1 hour 10 min	Muscles ached after yesterday – mustn't forget my stretches!

INTRODUCTION TO THE WORKOUTS

Make sure that if you have any medical or physical conditions which may affect your training programme you consult your GP before you begin the workouts.

You must start every workout with a short warm-up so the muscles you are about to use are relaxed, your joints are more mobile and your temperature and circulation have increased. If you are a complete beginner you may wish to start with the mobility exercises from the Pilates section (see page 98). After this I would recommend you do some stretching – holding the stretch for about 8 to 10 seconds – on all major muscle groups: quads, hamstrings, calves, hip flexors, chest, upper back (see pages 84–7). People who already do some exercise may find they don't need to stretch, and should just go straight on to do some cardiovascular work. Everyone should have a gradual cardiovascular warm-up of about 5 to 10 minutes (see page 106). You should notice your heart rate increasing, your breathing patterns begin to change, and your body's temperature begin to rise.

After a session I recommend you cool down gradually to bring the heart rate comfortably back to a normal level. Stretching is then a must for everyone! Repeat the warm-up stretches, aiming to develop the length of each muscle. These developmental stretches should be held for 30 to 45 seconds and are a way of calming the body and rounding off your workout. They should release tension as well as improve flexibility and prevent later muscular soreness from developing!

The workouts are designed so you can choose and vary your exercise regime. You may wish to begin with the general all-over toning workout on pages 112–21 which will work you top to toe. There are three levels to each exercise; remember to consider your body type and level of fitness when choosing the right one for you:

- ectomorphs should mainly work at Level 1
- mesomorphs should mainly work at Level 2
- endomorphs should mainly work at Level 3

Where weights are indicated in the workouts, start with light weights if you haven't done much exercise and use what suits you if you are already exercising. You should work your legs harder than your upper body, so if you use light hand weights, use medium leg weights. Don't stay at the same weight when you know you can increase the resistance – make sure you challenge yourself.

- light weights = 1–2 kg
- medium weights = 2–4 kg
- heavy weights = 5–10 kg

Repeat the workout a few times and, when you find it is becoming easier, make yourself work harder by increasing the weights you use, the number of repetitions or the amount of time you spend on each exercise.

STRETCHING

If you are a beginner you should do some stretches as part of your warm-up. If you are more advanced you may feel you don't need to do this, but stretching is an important part of your programme. In addition to using up calories, stretching lengthens your muscles and helps prevent injury. Do these stretches to cool down at the end of your session, too.

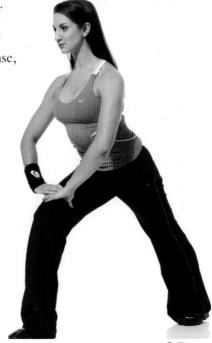

Quad Stretch

Stand on one foot and hold the other foot in your hand – hold on to something if you need to. Keep the knees soft. Draw the knee up and the foot back towards the spine until you feel a stretch in the front of the thigh. You can also do this stretch lying on one side with your knees bent up in line with the hips – hold the ankle of the top leg and, keeping the leg bent, draw it back so the knee is moving towards the spine. Stop when you get a stretch. Repeat on the other side. Hold the stretch for 30–45 seconds.

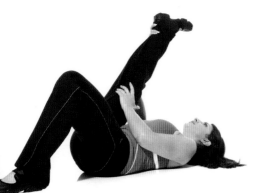

Hamstring Stretch

Lie on your back with knees bent, feet flat on the floor. Lift one leg and put one hand behind the knee (do NOT hold onto the kneecap) and the other hand behind your ankle. Straighten the leg until you feel a stretch at the back of the thigh. Try and ease the stretch a little further, release, and change legs. Hold the stretch for 30–45 seconds.

Calf Stretch

Stand with both hips and feet facing forwards. Step back with one foot, shift your weight forward so the front leg bends slightly and the upper body comes in line with the back leg. Keep the back heel down on the floor. You should feel the stretch in the back leg. Release and change legs. Hold the stretch for 30–45 seconds.

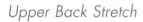

Upper Back Stretch

Clasp the hands in front of the body. Round the back, don't lock out the elbows, gently pull the arms forward and drop the chin to the chest. Hold the stretch for 10–15 seconds.

Triceps Stretch

Lift one arm and place the other hand on the elbow. Bend the arm so the hand is coming down between the shoulder blades. Gently push the arm back with the other hand until you feel a stretch in the back of the upper arm. Hold the stretch for 10–15 seconds. Or, take one arm across the body, put one hand just below the elbow and ease the arm further across. Release and change arms. Hold the stretch for 10–15 seconds.

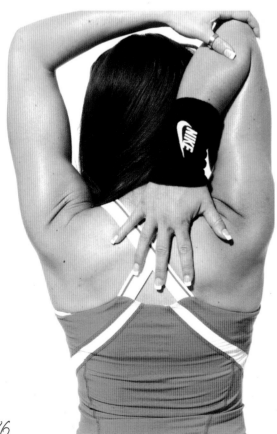

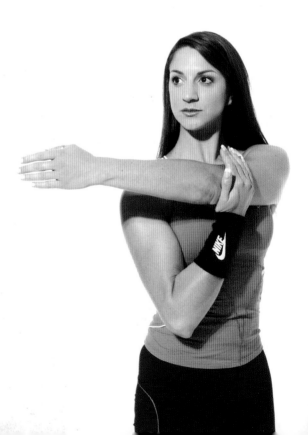

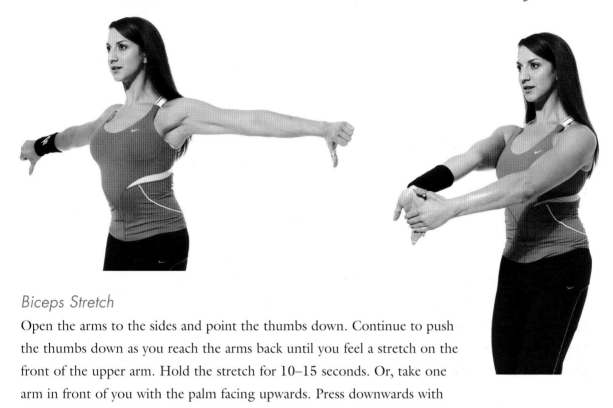

Biceps Stretch

Open the arms to the sides and point the thumbs down. Continue to push the thumbs down as you reach the arms back until you feel a stretch on the front of the upper arm. Hold the stretch for 10–15 seconds. Or, take one arm in front of you with the palm facing upwards. Press downwards with the other hand into the palm of the raised hand. Release and change arms. Hold the stretch for 10–15 seconds.

Chest Stretch

Place both hands in the small of the back. Keep the shoulders relaxed. Pull the elbows backwards until you feel a sufficient stretch across the chest. Hold the stretch for 10–15 seconds. Or, turn and face a wall and lift one arm to shoulder height. Place the hand on the wall and slowly turn the body away from the arm. Hold the stretch for 10–15 seconds.

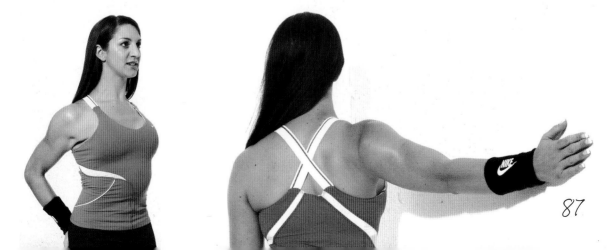

CORE TRAINING

Core stability is an essential part of our life, yet we often fail to realize the effect it has on our everyday activities. Without a stable core, your muscles are not optimally balanced, and your natural movement pattern will adapt to this imbalance which can lead to injury. Many people develop back pain as a result of weak or unused core muscles and that is why it is important to include specific exercises for this area. Core stability also improves balance, muscular co-ordination and the ability to develop power. Without building a good stable core you may not be able to reach your full potential in the rest of the programme.

Pelvic Stability

The first step to increase strength in the pelvic area involves establishing and recognizing a 'neutral position'. Once this position is in place you can apply small challenges to your centre with your levers (arms and legs) to make your core work harder in maintaining your stability.

Neutral Spine/Relaxation Position

- Lie on your back with your knees bent and feet flat on the floor hip-width apart.
- Begin to relax the body.
- Breathe in, then breathe out and release your shoulders. Let them soften, drop and open.
- Breathe in again and then breathe out and release your ribcage so it softens in to the floor.
- Continue breathing wide into your ribcage – as if breathing into the floor.
- Place the heels of your hands on the hip bones and fingers on the pubic bone (your hands form a diamond shape).

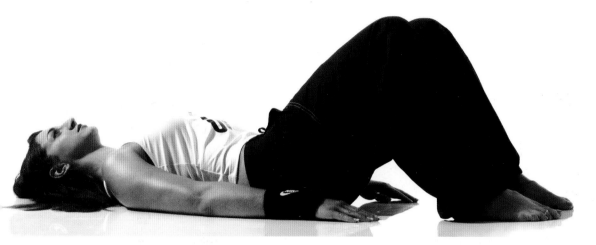

- Gently tilt the pelvis down and up until it feels as though your hands are parallel to the floor (not pointing down or up).
- Draw the navel towards the spine so it is contracted 30 per cent (draw the tummy slightly away from the hands).
- Maintain the breathing and continue to engage your abdominal muscles.

This position may not feel too difficult to hold, but you should have a constant sense of awareness in the neutral position. All movement should challenge this neutral and engaged position, which means that you may have to engage your abdominals to 70–80 per cent to avoid any unwanted movement in the pelvis or spine when performing the exercises at the most difficult phase.

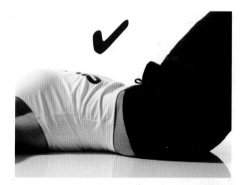

Synchronizing your breathing is not essential when you are doing these exercises so please do not feel overwhelmed if you cannot co-ordinate the breath with the movement straight away. Keep your breathing slow and controlled and in time you may wish to adjust your breathing to the movement. This will improve your overall focus and co-ordination.

Try the following exercises, repeating them a few times.

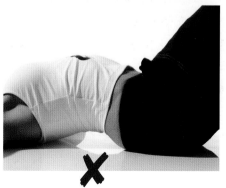

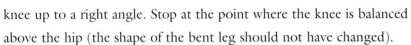

Knee Folds

- Get into neutral.
- Breathe in to prepare.
- Breathe out, engage navel to spine and slowly fold the right knee up to a right angle. Stop at the point where the knee is balanced above the hip (the shape of the bent leg should not have changed).
- Breathe wide into the ribcage (try to avoid any tension building with the breath).
- Breathe out and slowly return the bent leg back to the floor (make sure the abdominals do not dome or the back arch).
- Repeat with the left leg.

Knee Circles

You will need either a Dynaband, a pair of tights or a towel.

- Wrap the Dynaband around the back of one thigh close to the knee.
- Find neutral spine.
- Lift the right leg up to a right angle using the above technique for knee folds. Hold the band with the right hand and make sure the elbow is on the floor.
- Imagine you are drawing circles with your knee on the ceiling. Make sure there is no movement anywhere else in the body apart from the thigh bone rotating in the hip socket, pull navel to

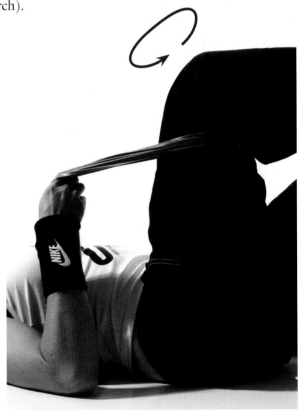

spine treating it like the centre pin of all your movement. There should be NO rocking at the pelvis.

- Breathe normally.
- Circle the knee in the opposite direction.
- Repeat on the other side.

Notice how much you have to pull in your stomach to maintain a neutral position – and there is hardly any movement from the body at this point!

Knee Drops

This is not a hip mobility exercise to see how far the knee can open, this is an exercise to see how far the knee can drop while keeping the hips level and the pelvis completely stable.

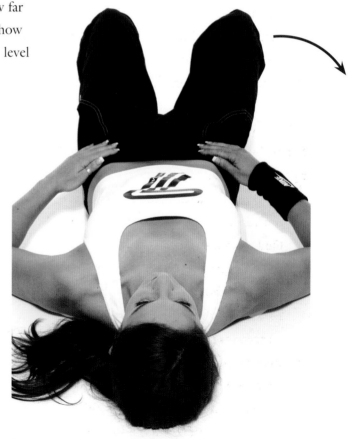

- Find neutral spine.
- Breathe in to prepare.
- Breathe out and allow one knee to fall to the side. Resist the weight of your leg as you keep control in your centre (do not let the opposite knee fall out as a counterbalance).
- Breathe in to hold.
- Breathe out and draw navel to spine to pull the knee back in to the starting position.
- Repeat with the opposite leg.

Imagine your centre is like a fishing rod. You are allowing the knee to drop under a slow release line and drawing the knee back in with control.

ABDOMINAL BUILDING

How many times have you done a sit-up to gain flat abs? Are you getting flat abs? As with posture, it's important to work the muscles the way we eventually want them to look. When you perform a sit-up it probably hurts, which means you are using the abdominals; if you touch the muscle, you can feel it has tensed. This indicates that the muscle has been activated and most people can actually see it tighten outwards. Hang on . . . if you can see the abdominal muscle tightening and contracting in a domed shape outwards, which way are you building the abdominal growth? Outwards!

If you want to have lengthened, toned, flatter abdominals it is critical you work the muscle inwards and keep it pulled in when performing any exercise. This can only be achieved with core strength and mastering the technique of engaging and drawing navel to spine in anticipation of any performed movement.

Contracting Navel to Spine

Here is the safest sit-up in the world. I guarantee you will be working the abdominals inwards without any of the pains and strains people often get when doing this movement incorrectly.

- Lie on the floor face down (take a few moments to relax).
- Place your head on your hands so you are comfortable.
- Breathe in.
- Breathe out and pull the navel into the spine to around 70 per cent of the maximum contraction you could achieve. Imagine there is a piece of cold ice underneath you and you're trying to lift away from it.
- Breathe in and hold the abdominals contracted (your new training point).
- Breathe out to relax.

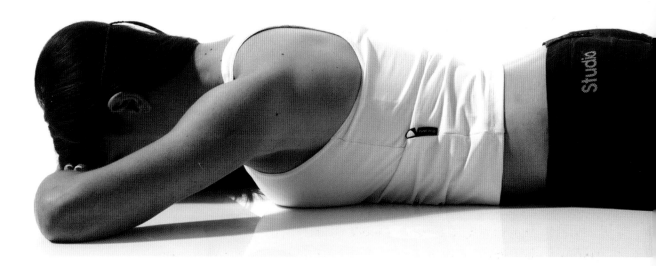

Repeat this at least 10 times and as often as you can so you feel comfortable with the process. The more you practise the easier it will become.

Once you have completed this exercise try holding the abdominals at the 70 per cent mark and continue breathing normally. Hold the contraction for around 10 to 30 seconds and then release. This will increase your ability to hold and sustain a contraction and will help you in later exercises.

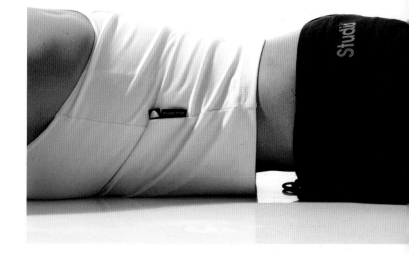

You may also want to try the same exercises on all fours which will let you see just how much you can pull in your abdominal area. Make sure you do not let the back arch when you lift or sink when you release.

Pelvic Floor

The pelvic floor muscle is the muscle responsible for holding the bladder, bowels and womb in place and closes the anus, vagina and urethra. Most people do not use this muscle enough which means it becomes lazy and lax. Women are often taught exercises to re-tighten this muscle after they have given birth, but it is sometimes hard to feel because it is weak and possibly damaged.

The pelvic floor muscle is the one you would squeeze to stop in mid flow when you are passing water. Now, although this is a great way to understand where the pelvic floor is I wouldn't advise you to go running off to the loo to practise as this can actually weaken the muscle as opposed to strengthening it.

Here's what I want you to do to strengthen and improve the use of your pelvic floor:

- Sit cross-legged (or have feet quite far from your bottom with the soles together if that's more comfortable) grow tall and straight (no slouching!).
- Put your hands underneath your bottom, palms up and fingers spread wide, so you can feel the base of your spine.
- Squeeze your bottom and feel how you lift off your hands as the muscles contract, then relax.
- Squeeze the muscle in the space between your hands and fingertips (between both buttocks), draw up and in with the contraction. Try and hold it before you release.

Once you have tried that a few times and have established where the muscle is, try the following exercise while seated, to focus and improve the contraction:

- Imagine the pelvic floor is like a lift waiting at ground level.
- Close the lift doors and squeeze up to the first floor.
- Hold the contraction, then take the lift back to the ground floor and release the doors.

- Close the doors again and take the lift to the first floor, hold here and then squeeze up to the second floor, hold, then release back to ground level.

Repeat as many times as you want and as often as you want; remember, no one can ever see you working your pelvic floor because it's all on the inside! While performing the pelvic floor exercise try to avoid squeezing your buttocks and legs or pulling your stomach in. Make sure you don't hold your breath!

INTRODUCTION TO PILATES WORKOUT

I once read about the slow process of Pilates and how it can have the power to change your posture and life forever. Joseph Pilates said:

- up to 10 sessions to feel the difference
- up to 20 sessions to see the difference
- up to 30 sessions to have a whole new body

I have given you this Pilates warm-up and mini workout for those of you who are short of time or who want a less strenuous workout. You can incorporate the pelvic stability exercises described above into this workout to increase the length. This is also a useful workout to add into your exercise programme because it will stretch and tone your muscles at the same time as making sure you are using your body in a good way.

However, if you want to get active and out there, feel free to skip to the section that suits you best. This book is not a military step-by-step process; it's all about choices that are right for you, making this an enjoyable experience and an ongoing journey.

MOBILITY WARM-UP

It is important to make sure the body has a gentle pulse-raiser and mobility warm-up for Pilates. Follow these suggested exercises because you will be stretching and lengthening the muscles during the programme and want to maximize the benefits.

Breathing

Stand in a neutral position (see Correct Alignment Checklist on page 195), breathe in and take the arms out to the sides allowing your ribcage to open laterally. Then breathe out, releasing the arms back down and softening the ribcage. Repeat as many times as you need to energize your body. Then inhale, take the arms over the head and stretch, feeling the abdominals lengthen. Take care not to arch the back. Exhale and release the arms back down. Repeat 5 times.

Head Mobility

Stand in neutral (see page 195) and look straight ahead, then look down at your chest. Bring the head back up. Turn your head to the right; bring it back to centre. Turn your head to the left; bring it back to centre. Tilt the head down to the right shoulder; bring it back to centre, then tilt down to the left shoulder and come back to centre.

Ankle Circles

Stand in neutral (see page 195) on one leg with the knee lifted in front of you and at hip height, with the toe pointing downwards (hold on to a surface if you need to). Circle the ankle in one direction 5 times, then in the other direction 5 times. Try just to work in the ankle joint, don't move the leg. Repeat with the other leg. This should help improve your balance and mobility at the same time.

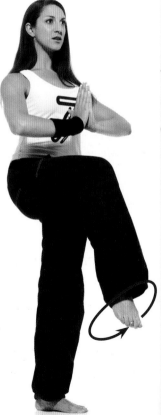

Angel Wings

Inhale, then exhale and lift the arms out to the sides, bend the elbows and put the fingertips on the back of the head. Inhale and lift the shoulders, exhale and let the shoulders drop, inhale and take the elbows back – without sticking the ribcage out or arching your back – exhale and stretch the arms out to the sides and lower. Repeat 5 times.

Swinging Down and Up

Standing in a neutral position (see page 195), breathe in and lift the arms above the head. Breathe out, bend the knees and swing the arms down and behind you. Breathe in as you swing the arms back up above the head, straightening the knees at the same time – avoid arching the back as you reach up. Repeat 10 times.

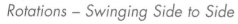

Rotations – Swinging Side to Side

Stand with your feet hip-width apart and your arms raised to shoulder level, and swing from side to side, letting your body turn easily and lifting the heel of the foot you are turning away from to avoid twisting the knee. Look in the direction you are turning so you are looking slightly over your shoulder.

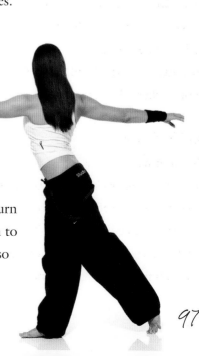

PILATES MINI WORKOUT

Roll Down into Press-Up

Start from neutral spine (see page 195) with feet and hips shoulder-distance apart. Breathe in then breathe out, navel to spine, and roll the head, shoulders and upper body down as if peeling away from a Velcro wall. Do NOT lean back on the heels or send the bottom out. Aim your weight slightly forward, keeping the knees soft. Roll all the way down, bending the knees as much as you need, and walk out on the hands (resting on your knees if preferred) keeping the abdominals pulled in and the hips level. Make sure the hands are wider than the shoulders and do a press-up, making sure you engage navel to spine.

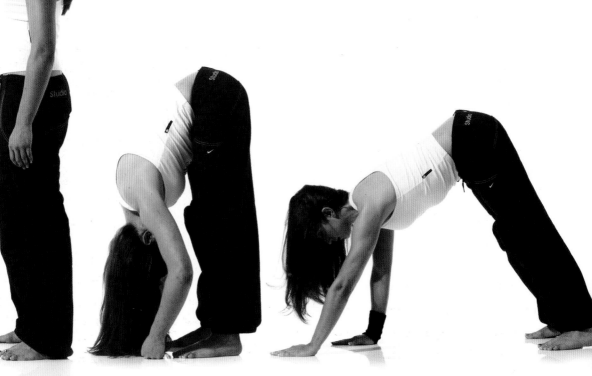

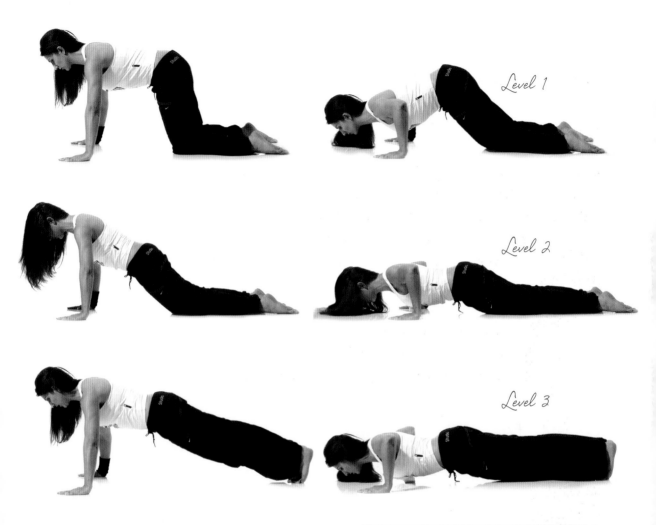

Level 1

Level 2

Level 3

- Level 1 do a box press-up (head in front of hands)
- Level 2 do a half press-up (take the bottom in line with the spine)
- Level 3 do a full press-up (take the knees away from the floor)

Breathe in then breathe out as you roll back up through the vertebrae – imagining you are building blocks through your spine one on top of the other – make sure the head is the last thing to lift up.

SETS: 1
REPS LEVEL 1: 8-15 box press-ups
      LEVEL 2: 8-15 half press-ups
      LEVEL 3: 8-15 full press-ups
DEVELOPMENT:
- Do a full press-up, then lift one leg keeping the hips level, hold for 5-10 seconds before lowering and returning.
- Do a full press-up with one leg raised.
INCREASES: mobility and strength

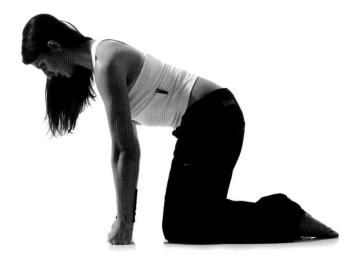

Cat Stretch

Start on all fours, hands directly under your shoulders, knees directly under your hips, in neutral. Breathe in then breathe out and tuck the head and tailbone down to the floor as you pull up through the centre of the back and stretch. Slowly release and allow the back to give a little in the opposite direction but not too much.

SETS: 1
REPS LEVEL 1: 4-6
LEVEL 2: 6-8
LEVEL 3: 8-10
INCREASES: mobility

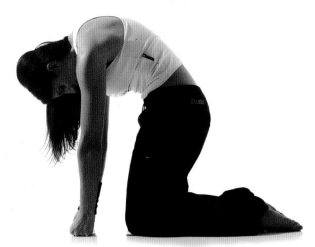

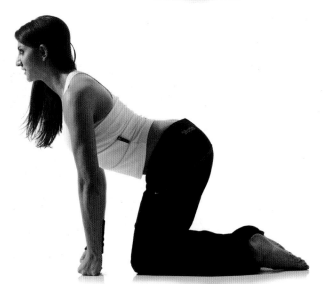

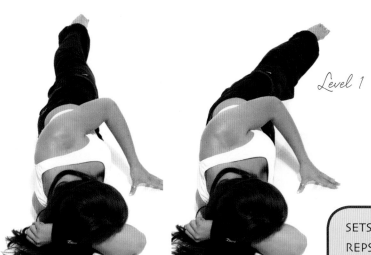

Level 1

SETS: 1
REPS LEVEL 1: 4-6
LEVEL 2: 6-8
LEVEL 3: 8-10
DEVELOPMENT:
• Lift both legs and perform a scissor action – top leg slightly forward, lower leg slightly back, then alternate legs keeping the alignment of the body.
INCREASES: strength and mobility

Side Kick

Lie on one side in a straight line with your hips and shoulders stacked on top of each other. Bring the feet and legs slightly forward so if you look down you should be able to see your toes. Bend one arm to rest the head on to avoid neck tension. Place the fingertips of the other hand in front of you to aid your balance. Don't rock forward or backward. Engage navel to spine.

- Level 1 – breathe in and lift the top leg to hip level, then breathe out as you take the top leg forward. Do not let the hips fall forward, only take the leg as far forward as you can remain stable and feel a challenge on the abdominal area. Breathe in to return (keep the leg at hip height throughout the exercise).
- Level 2 – lift both legs and perform the above exercise.
- Level 3 – as Level 2, but take the supporting hand away to reduce the stability.

Repeat on the other side.

Level 2

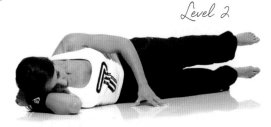

Level 3

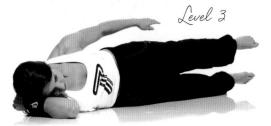

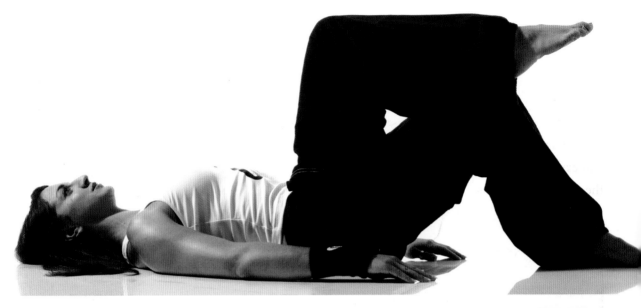

Knee Folds

You will breathe out on all the movements for this exercise. Lie on your back on the floor in neutral spine (see page 88) with knees bent and feet hip-width apart. Breathe in to prepare. Breathe out, engage navel to spine and slowly fold the right knee up at a right angle and stop at the point where the knee is balanced above the hip (the shape of the bent leg should not have changed). Breathe in wide through the ribcage (try and avoid any tension building with the breath). Breathe out and slowly return the foot to the floor (make sure the abdominals do not dome or the back arch). Repeat with the left leg.

SETS: 1
REPS LEVEL 1: 4-6
     LEVEL 2: 6-8
     LEVEL 3: 8-10
DEVELOPMENT:
- Double knee folds – lift the first leg, then the second leg. Lower the first leg, then the second leg.
- Start with both legs lifted then lower one leg until the tips of the toes reach the floor and then lift back up while the opposite leg is lowering.
INCREASES: strength

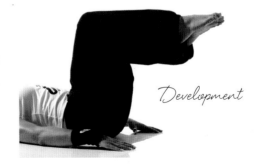

Development

Single Leg Extension

Lie on the back in a double knee fold (see opposite page). Breathe in to prepare. Breathe out, contract navel to spine as you extend one leg away – do NOT allow the back to arch or the abdominals to dome. Breathe in as you return knee at a right angle then repeat on the opposite side.

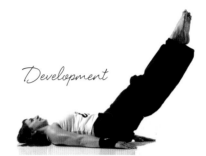

Development

SETS: 1

REPS LEVEL 1: 4-6

       LEVEL 2: 6-8

       LEVEL 3: 8-10

DEVELOPMENT:

- Extend one leg and as the leg retracts extend the other leg.
- Extend both legs together, then retract, maintaining strong neutral spine. Don't let the back arch.
- Lower legs slowly, as close to the floor as your strength allows.

TIP: lengthen out to stretch

INCREASES: strength

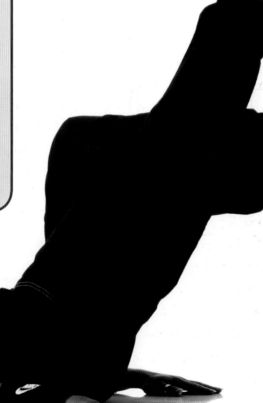

Shoulder Bridge

Lie on the floor on your back in neutral spine. Breathe in then breathe out and pull navel to spine. Allow the pelvis to tilt and begin to peel the spine away from the floor (notch by notch as if peeling away from a tacky surface). Take the position as high as you feel comfortable, but no higher than the shoulder blades. Breathe in to hold. Breathe out as you lower down slowly, one vertebra at a time, aiming to stretch the spine as you lower. Come back to neutral spine.

SETS: 1
REPS LEVEL 1: 4-6
LEVEL 2: 6-8
LEVEL 3: 8-10
DEVELOPMENT:
- Once in the bridge position lift both arms up and over head so they touch the floor; as you lower the body allow the arms to return back to sides.
- Once in the bridge position extend one leg, keeping the hips and knees in line. Lower the spine back to the floor with the leg still lifted, keeping hips level. When you are down draw the leg back in.

INCREASES: mobility and strength

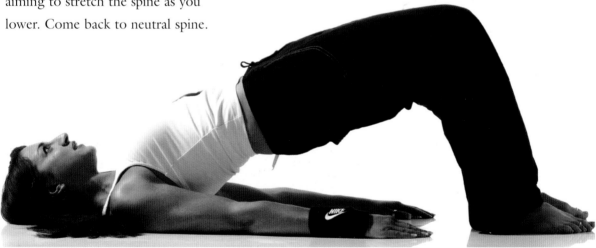

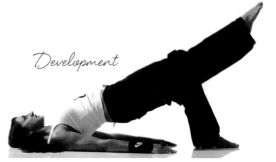

Development

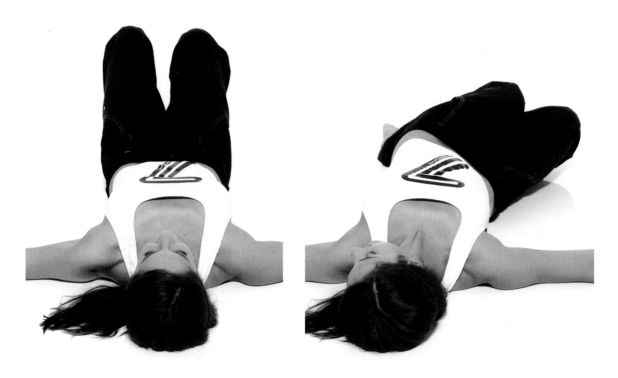

Hip Rolls

Lie on the floor on your back in neutral spine, legs together, arms out to the sides, palms facing up. Breathe in to prepare. Breathe out, navel to spine, and allow your legs to drop to one side with control while your head rolls the other way. Breathe in, to prepare for the return. Breathe out, engage the abdominals and return the knees back to centre aiming to pull the knees back with the strength of the abdominal contraction.

SETS: 1
REPS LEVEL 1: 4-6
        LEVEL 2: 6-8
        LEVEL 3: 8-10
DEVELOPMENT:
- Start with both legs lifted, keep the knees together and extend one leg, then roll towards the bent knee. Repeat on the same side for a set and then change legs and direction.
INCREASES: mobility

CARDIOVASCULAR WARM-UP AND OUTDOOR WORKOUT

You should always do some cardiovascular work as part of your warm-up: walking on the spot, skipping, doing some step work on the stairs, or you may have cardiovascular equipment you can use at home. You should work at a brisk pace and intensity – just hard enough to feel a gradual warming throughout the body. Alternatively, you can head outside for a walk or run (see page 110 for tips on walking and running) and keep a mild pace until you have reached a point where it feels comfortable to begin your main workout.

The following walking and running workouts are suggestions of how to incorporate a bit more cardiovascular work into everyday life. Remember you should try to spend 20 to 60 minutes on cardiovascular activity three to five times a week.

If you are just starting to exercise, you should think of starting at the beginners level walking, then progress to intermediate and advanced and then go on to the running programme (see page 109). Even if you are advanced they should provide some useful tips on how to walk and run correctly, and you can decide if you would like to incorporate the programmes into your daily routine.

Walking Workout

Walking is a great way to improve your cardiovascular fitness, burn fat and lower your blood pressure. It will also help improve your muscle tone and strengthen your bones while being joint friendly with no impact. You can walk anywhere on any surface – hills can vary your programme and increase intensity, for example. There is no equipment required except a good pair of trainers to support and cushion your feet and comfortable clothing that suits the weather. You can begin walking immediately.

Keep your route simple to begin with and in a public area (in case you feel ill). In a less public area you should equip yourself with a mobile phone and let people know you are going out. If you plan to walk in the country take a map, phone or whistle, and for any journey take fluids to quench your thirst and stay hydrated. As you increase the time and distance, start to vary your routes to make it more interesting.

Although you have walked for the majority of your life, walking for cardiovascular exercise should be different to your everyday stroll. You should walk with more precision and effort. Progress to intermediate when you have performed a few walks at beginner's level and feel ready.

Walking: Beginner

- Walk with a purpose – stride out further than usual.
- Bring the heels down first.
- Swing the arms straight and from the shoulders as opposed to across body, thumbs should point in the direction of travel.
- Look up and to the front.
- Squeeze the gluteals to power forward.

Walking: Intermediate and Advanced

In order to progress (i.e. speed up your pace) you need to adopt these techniques:

- Increase the pace by lifting the toes higher, revealing the sole of the shoe.
- Drive back with slightly bent elbows for more power.
- Push from the gluteals.

Get your walking technique right because when you progress to a running programme you will be striking the floor with much greater force. It's important your technique is correct to avoid any injuries.

Walking Workout

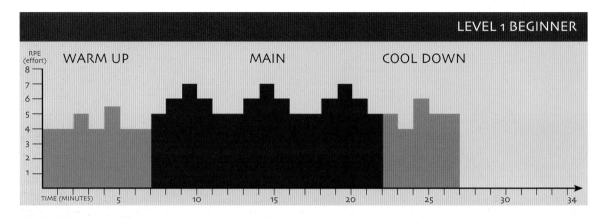

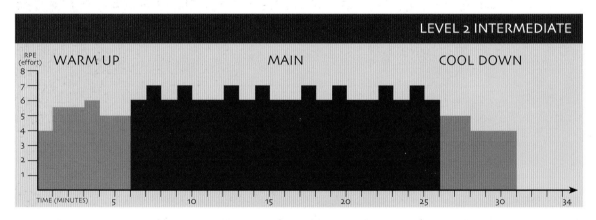

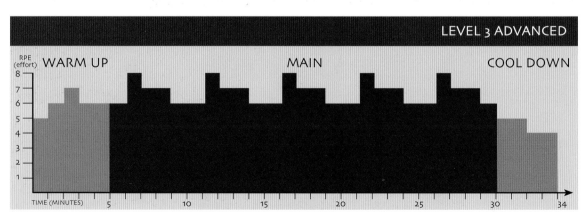

Running Programme

This is a 6-week programme that gets progressively harder to challenge you further as you get fitter. Intersperse the running with a recovery period where you walk fast.

Week	Running (minutes)	Recovery: fast walk (minutes)	Reps	Per week	Total time
1	3	3	4	2–3	24 mins
2	4	3	4	2–3	28 mins
3	4	2.5	4	2–3	26 mins
4	4	2	5	2–3	30 mins
5	5	1.5	5	2–3	32.5 mins
6	5–6	1	5	2–3	30–35 mins

After 6 weeks increase your running time and have a recovery time of between 1 and 3 minutes as needed. Progress further by reducing your recovery time until you do not need it at all. Remember to stretch calf, hip flexors, hamstrings and quads for 10 to 15 seconds after the warm up and for 30 to 45 seconds after the cool down.

Tips on How to Walk and Run

- Walk or run in a 'heel, ball, toe' action. Strike the floor with the heel and transfer the weight through the back of the foot and push off for the next step from the toe.
- Keep your arms relaxed at a 90° angle rather than letting them swing by your sides. The shoulders should swing slightly forward and backward without rounding. Keep the body and hips facing forward.
- If there's an incline, increase your speed to challenge yourself.
- Drive your legs from the gluteals (see glossary, page 216), lifting the toes, and use the arms to propel you forward. Aim to push off the back leg.
- When walking uphill take smaller strides and try looking slightly down to make the ground appear flat rather than seeing the hill ahead. Lean into the hill slightly from the hips to aid your action and engage your abdominals. When walking downhill engage your abdominals slightly, bend the knees a little and lean back to help control movement.
- Keep your head up and walk tall. Inhale fully and deeply, then exhale fully; try to regulate your breathing with your stride. Quicker, smaller steps will take you further than long ones, however, longer strides will allow more stretch in the hips – aim to work with smaller steps but take some long strides towards the end of the walk to cool down.
- Don't cross the arms in front of your chest as this can interfere with your breathing.
- Make sure you are sufficiently hydrated before your walk or run.
- Do not run on a full or empty stomach.
- Invest in decent trainers for stability and joint support. Change your trainers approximately every 4 to 6 months.

Now it's time to get started with the cardiovascular work. I have given you a selection of things to do – some are static and repetitive (for those who prefer a structured non-mind-challenging approach) and some routine (for those who like to challenge the mind and enjoy variety). Please feel free to adapt them or develop your own ideas! The total aerobic content of your workout should last 30 minutes which also includes a 5–10 minute gradual warm-up. A beginner new to exercise should aim to complete 20 minutes and increase the time gradually. As you improve and begin to vary your exercise regime, cardiovascular exercise can be increased to suit your work-out session. For example, if you are doing the circuit programme (see page 168) which contains cardiovascular intervals you may find that the warm-up plus the workout is enough. If you are doing the general toning workout (see page 122) you may add on a further 25 to 30 minutes of cardiovascular work. On the other hand you may wish to spend a session totally focusing on cardiovascular work for up to 60 minutes and not do any cardiovascular work (apart from warming up) the day before or the day following. Go back and look at the rate of perceived exertion scale (page 80) and aim to be work-ing in the 6–8 rating (able to say a few words but not hold a conversation!) or record your effort level when first starting out and see if it decreases as you improve. Then progress by increasing the intensity of your activity and continue recording your performance (remember these may vary depending on the time of day you exercise).

 Although the programme is flexible try to put it in your diary to ensure it becomes and stays part of the new you.

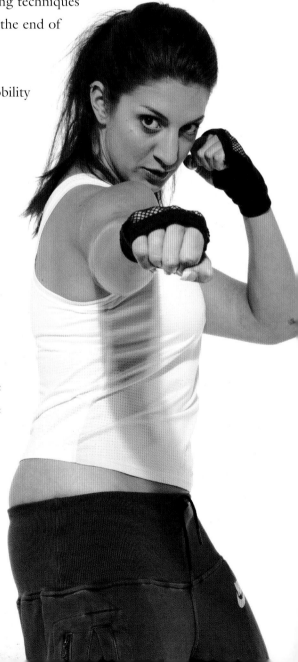

WORKOUT ONE
AEROBIC

You will need to learn the correct punching and kicking techniques for these exercises – a great way to vent frustration at the end of a tough day!

Warm-up: 5 minutes – includes stretching and mobility (see pages 84–7 and 96–7)

PUNCHING TECHNIQUE

Starting position: if you are right handed step back with your right leg, with the foot slightly turned out and the knees soft. Your hips and torso will be facing towards the right. If you are left handed reverse the foot and leg position.

On guard: fists clenched facing inwards, with the thumb on top of the fist, next to the cheeks and close to the chin. Tuck the chin down slightly and keep the elbows in.

Jab: rotate while pushing the right arm out from the shoulder so the torso slightly turns clockwise (left arm and anti-clockwise if you are left handed). Do not lock the elbow. This is a quick punch in front of you. Return to the on-guard position.

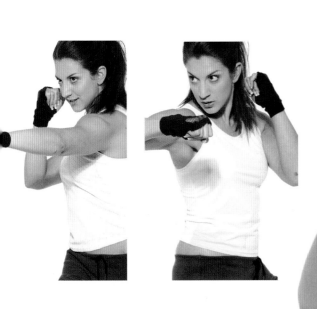

Cross: the same technique as a jab but the arm comes across the body and the back heel swivels to face forward as do the hips. Combining a jab and a cross is called the 1–2 combination.

Hook: drop at the knees and swing the fist slightly outwards to swing across the front of the body, aiming to have contact with your opponent's cheek. The elbow is lifted so it is in line with the wrist. Release the heels and rotate the torso as you swing. Engage the abdominals for power.

Uppercut: drop at the knees and bring the elbow down to the hip. Strike the fist forward and upward in front of the body aiming to hit your opponent's chin. When performing an uppercut with the back arm release the heel and face the hips forward.

The first section of the workout takes place indoors.

Step-ups
Using the stairs and alternating legs, step up, up, down, down.
Time: optional

Skipping Combo
You don't even need a skipping rope for this, you can just imagine it as you skip!

- heel to bottom x 8
- travel forward 8 steps x 4
- on the spot x 8
- travel back 8 steps x 4

Time: approx. 5 minutes

Boxing Combo
Jacks – jump out with both feet, keeping the knees soft and in line with the toes. Lift the arms out to the sides at the same time. Jump back to the starting position and lower the arms.

Half jacks – step to the side with the right foot and put your body weight on the right leg. At the same time, lift both arms to the sides. Bring the foot and arms back to the starting position. Do these with the same arm and then repeat on the other side.

- jabs x 8, jacks or half jacks x 8   repeat 4 times
- jabs x 4, jacks or half jacks x 4   repeat 4 times
- jabs x 2, jacks or half jacks x 2   repeat 4 times
- jabs x 1, jacks or half jacks x 1   repeat 4 times

Time: approx. 5 minutes

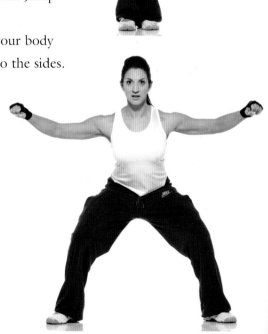

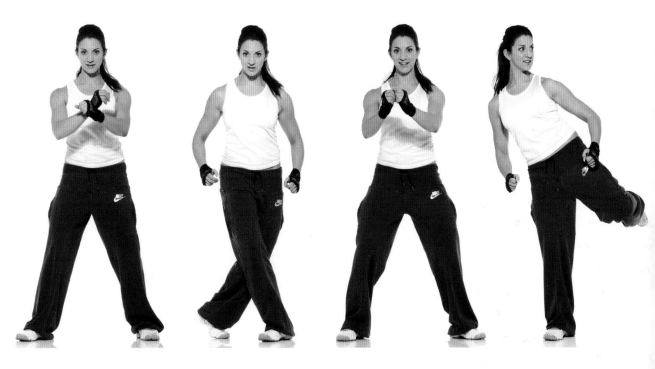

Grapevines and Leg Curls

Leg curls are performed by lightly kicking the heel in towards the bottom. In this exercise you will be moving sideways.

Step to the right, left foot behind right, step to the right, leg curl with the left leg, place the foot on the floor to the left, right foot behind the left, step to the left, leg curl with the right leg. Repeat.

Time: optional

Grapevine and Knee Lift

In this exercise you will be moving sideways and lifting the knee up towards the hip.

Step to the right, left foot behind the right, knee lift with the left leg, replace the foot on the floor to the left, right foot behind the left, knee lift with the right leg. Repeat.

Time: optional

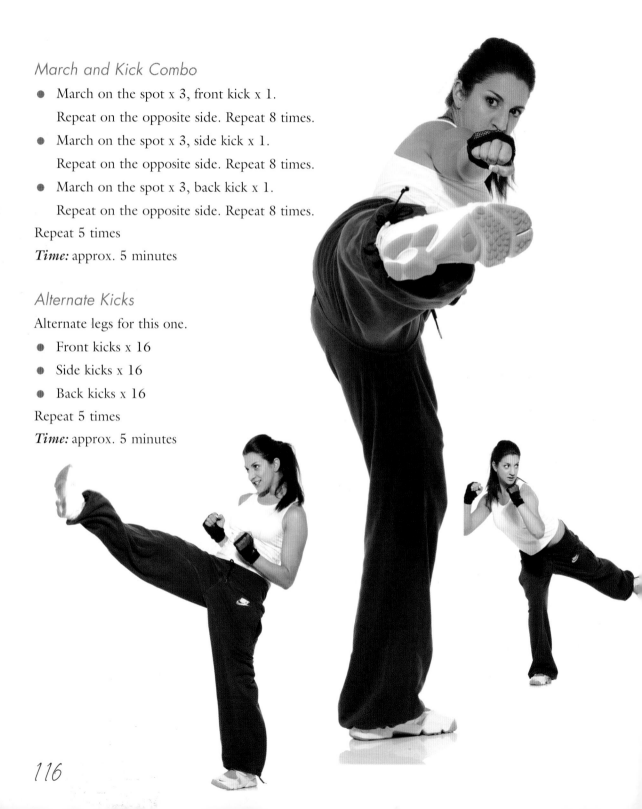

March and Kick Combo

- March on the spot x 3, front kick x 1.
  Repeat on the opposite side. Repeat 8 times.
- March on the spot x 3, side kick x 1.
  Repeat on the opposite side. Repeat 8 times.
- March on the spot x 3, back kick x 1.
  Repeat on the opposite side. Repeat 8 times.

Repeat 5 times

Time: approx. 5 minutes

Alternate Kicks

Alternate legs for this one.

- Front kicks x 16
- Side kicks x 16
- Back kicks x 16

Repeat 5 times

Time: approx. 5 minutes

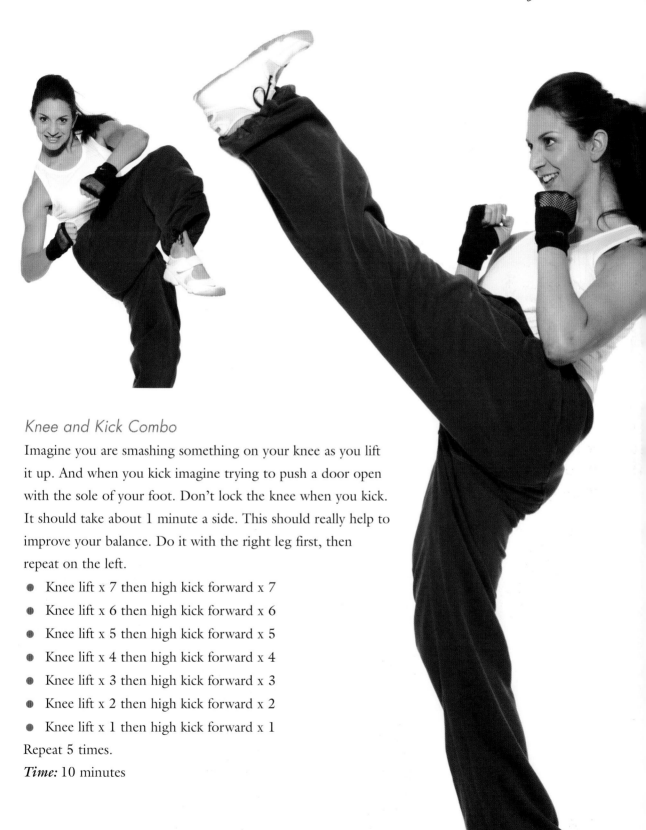

Knee and Kick Combo

Imagine you are smashing something on your knee as you lift
it up. And when you kick imagine trying to push a door open
with the sole of your foot. Don't lock the knee when you kick.
It should take about 1 minute a side. This should really help to
improve your balance. Do it with the right leg first, then
repeat on the left.

- Knee lift x 7 then high kick forward x 7
- Knee lift x 6 then high kick forward x 6
- Knee lift x 5 then high kick forward x 5
- Knee lift x 4 then high kick forward x 4
- Knee lift x 3 then high kick forward x 3
- Knee lift x 2 then high kick forward x 2
- Knee lift x 1 then high kick forward x 1

Repeat 5 times.

Time: 10 minutes

Knee Lifts

Standing on the spot, lift the knees alternately.

Time: optional

Side Step

Step to the side with your right foot, touch the left foot to the right, then step to the side with the left foot and touch the right foot to the left.

Time: optional

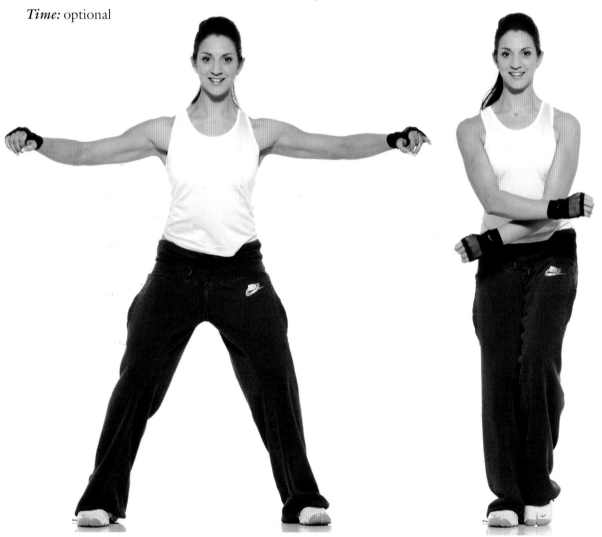

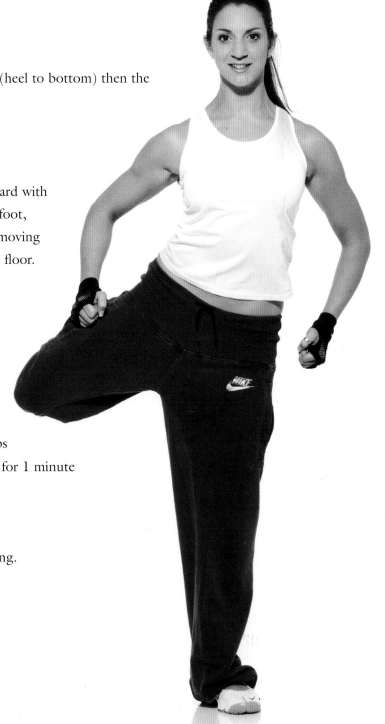

Leg Curls

Standing on the spot, curl the left leg (heel to bottom) then the right leg (heel to bottom). Repeat.
Time: optional

Easy Walk

Step forward with the right foot, forward with the left. Step backward with the right foot, then backward with the left. Imagine moving forward and backward in a box on the floor.
Time: optional

Skipping Circuit
(with or without rope)

- Skipping for 1 minute or 60 skips
- Jabs x 8, hooks x 8, uppercuts x 8 for 1 minute
- Skipping for 2 minutes or 120 skips
- Jabs x 8, hooks x 8, uppercuts x 8 for 1 minute

Time: 5 minutes

Rope Skipping

Breathe comfortably while rope skipping.
Time: optional

Now you've completed the indoor section of the workout, you can go and get some fresh air!

15-Minute Walk/Jog

This should be done at a brisk pace and you should aim to reach the level of RPE indicated in brackets (see page 80 for the RPE scale).

LEVEL ONE

- 2-minute walk (6)
- 2-minute walk (6)
- 2-minute walk (6)
- 2-minute walk (6)
- 2-minute walk (6)

- 1-minute jog (7)
- 1-minute jog (7)
- 1-minute jog (7)
- 1-minute jog (7)
- 1-minute jog (7)

For Level 2 walk for one minute and jog for 2 minutes.

For Level 3 walk for one minute and jog for 3 minutes.

As you continue to develop increase the jogging and reduce the walking.

Cardiovascular Activity with Equipment

If you have cardiovascular equipment, i.e. a rower or a bicycle at home, you may wish to do the following using a scale of 1–10 where 1 is the lowest amount of effort and 10 the highest. Choose a level and work for 10 to 20 minutes at an intensity that will maintain or challenge this level.

One of the best ways to lose fat and improve your cardiovascular capabilities is to mix periods of high effort and intensity with a period of recovery. I have therefore suggested three different programmes at different levels of intensity. As you improve, the intensity and length of time will have to be increased to maintain your workout effort level. This type of training is more demanding than lower intensity, but the extra effort will make for speedier changes and benefits!

LEVEL 1

- 1 minute at high intensity at Level 8
- 1 minute of recovery at Level 5

Repeat 5 times

Time: 10 minutes

LEVEL 2

- 2-minute warm-up
- 3 minutes at Level 5
- 3 minutes at Level 7
- 3 minutes at Level 9 – repeat this 2–3 times
- 3 minutes at Level 5

Cool down 2–4 minutes

Time: about 19–24 minutes

LEVEL 3

2-minute warm-up

Start at a low level and increase the intensity of effort each minute
until your maximum personal effort is reached, then decrease the effort
every minute.

Time: 20 minutes

Finish with the stretches on pages 84–7.

WORKOUT TWO
CONDITIONING AND ALL–OVER TONING

Hand weights are used for many of these exercises and you can make them at home by using two water-filled bottles or, to make them heavier, fill an empty bottle with sugar to the required weight.

Warm-up: 5 minutes stretching/mobility (see pages 84–7 and 96–7); 10–20 minutes cardiovascular activity (see pages 106–111)

Wide Squats

Stand with the feet slightly wider than the hips and the knees in line with the second toe. Keep the weight in the heels and think of the chest lifting as you bend the knees, then send the tailbone (the last bone in your spine) backwards while maintaining a flat back. Breathe out as you return to standing, slightly squeezing the abdominals and gluteals as you lift the body.

SETS: 2
REST PERIOD BETWEEN SETS: 30–60 seconds
REPS LEVEL 1: 10–12
      LEVEL 2: 12–15
      LEVEL 3: 15–20
DEVELOPMENT:
• Use hand weights.
• Stand on one leg.
MUSCLES WORKED: quads, gluteals, hamstrings

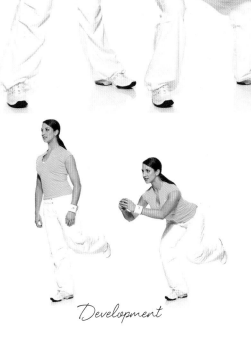

Development

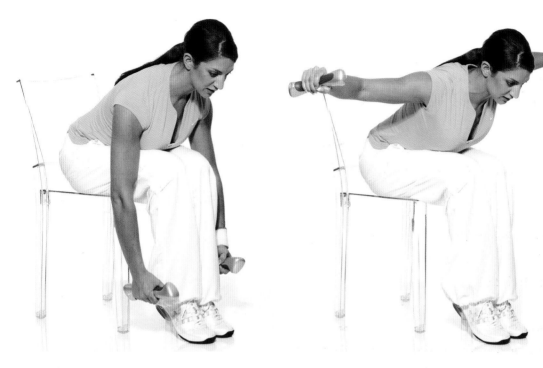

Seated Reverse Flies

Sit on a chair, leaning forward from the hips, with arms lengthening down
to the floor and palms facing inwards. Holding a weight in each hand,
lift the arms out to the sides to shoulder height, nip the shoulder blades
together, then return the arms to the sides.

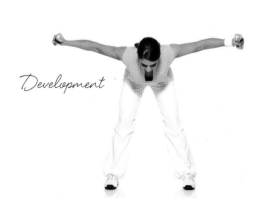

Development

SETS: 2
REST PERIOD BETWEEN SETS: 30–60 seconds
REPS LEVEL 1: 10–12
        LEVEL 2: 12–15
        LEVEL 3: 15–20
DEVELOPMENT:
• Increase the weight.
• Perform standing by engaging the
  abdominals, leaning forward from the hip
  and keeping the back straight.
MUSCLES WORKED: upper back

SETS: 2
REST PERIOD BETWEEN SETS: 30–60 seconds
REPS LEVEL 1: 10–12
         LEVEL 2: 12–15
         LEVEL 3: 15–20
DEVELOPMENT:
• Full press-up
MUSCLES WORKED: chest, triceps, abdominals

Press-Ups

Start on all fours, with your hands directly under your shoulders, fingers pointing forwards. Engage your abdominals and push your body weight into your hands, bending the elbows, to lower the upper body in a straight line from the hips down to the floor. Push the hands into the floor to lift the body back up. A full press-up is one with the legs stretched out behind you and toes tucked underneath.

Development

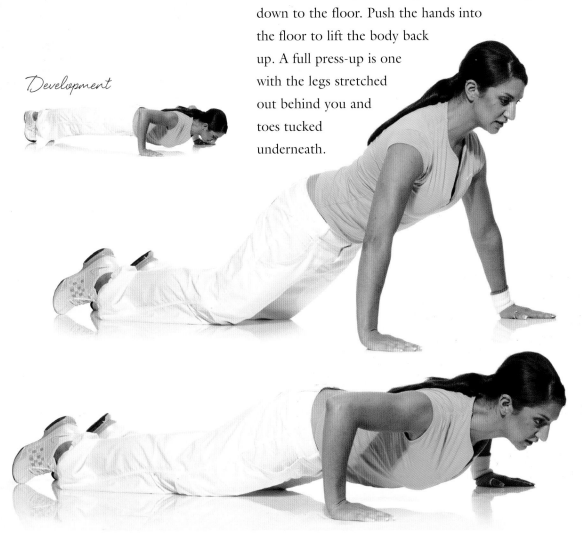

Weighted Shoulder Press

Start with a weight in each hand and arms at shoulder height.
Keep the elbows underneath the wrists. Push the weights up
above the head but slightly in front (so you can see your hands at
all times), don't lock the elbows. Return to the starting position.

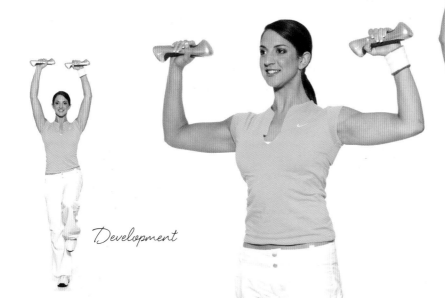

Development

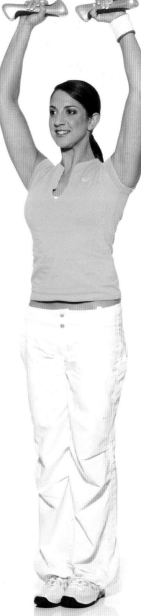

SETS: 2

REST PERIOD BETWEEN SETS: 30–60 seconds

REPS LEVEL 1: 10–12

LEVEL 2: 12–15

LEVEL 3: 15–20

DEVELOPMENT:

- Increase the weight.
- Perform standing on one leg.

MUSCLES WORKED: shoulders

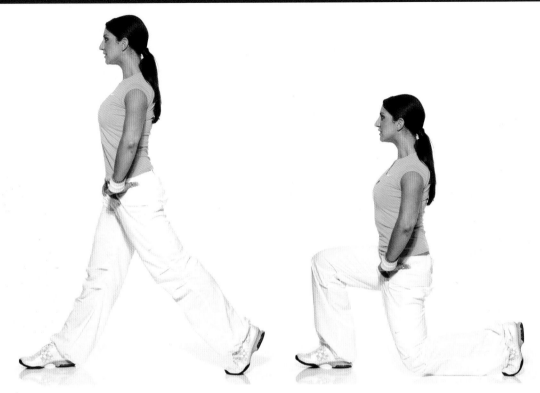

Lunges

Stand with feet hip-width apart, with one foot forward and one back. Lift the heel of the back foot. Lower the body down (not forwards) until you adopt a right angle with the back knee (your front knee should bend so your knee is above the ankle – NOT over the toe). Straighten back to the starting position.

SETS: 2

REST PERIOD BETWEEN SETS: 30–60 seconds

REPS LEVEL 1: 10–12

      LEVEL 2: 12–15

      LEVEL 3: 15–20

DEVELOPMENT:

- Make the lunges a non-stop pulsing action.
- Don't come all the way to the top before lowering back down.
- Perform the lunges at a much slower, controlled pace.
- Raise your arms in front of you for the lunge.

MUSCLES WORKED: quads, hamstrings, gluteals

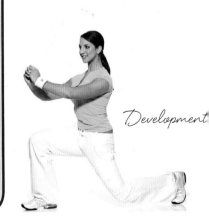

Development

Biceps Curl

Stand with your feet
shoulder-distance apart, with
a weight in each hand and
your arms by your sides.
Your hands should face
forward. Keep the elbows in
to the sides, bending them
to lift the weights. Do not
swing the trunk as you lift.
Lower the arms back to the
sides. Keep the elbows soft.

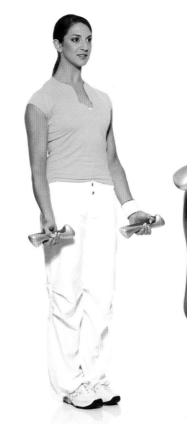

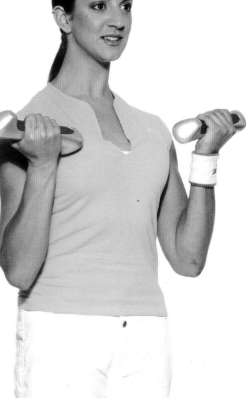

SETS: 2
REST PERIOD BETWEEN SETS:
   30–60 seconds
REPS LEVEL 1: 10–12
       LEVEL 2: 12–15
       LEVEL 3: 15–20
DEVELOPMENT:
- Increase the weight.
- Perform standing on one leg.
MUSCLES WORKED: biceps

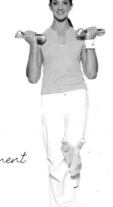

Development

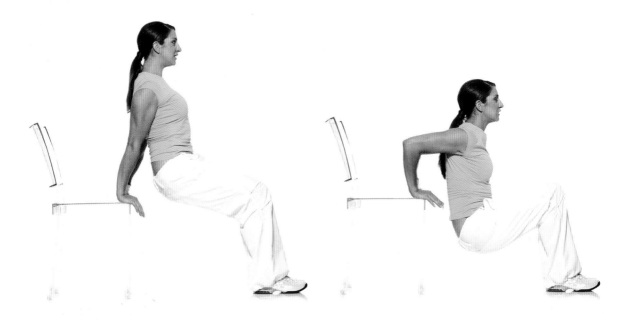

SETS: 2
REST PERIOD BETWEEN SETS: 30–60 seconds
REPS LEVEL 1: 10–12
        LEVEL 2: 12–15
        LEVEL 3: 15–20
DEVELOPMENT:
- Take the legs further away or straighten.
- Cross one leg over the other.
- Change position halfway through.
MUSCLES WORKED: triceps

Triceps Dips

Place a chair against a wall and sit on it with your knees bent and feet hip-distance apart. Have your hands on the edge of the chair with the fingers pointing forward. Straighten the arms to lift the bottom up away from the chair. Bend the elbows directly behind you to lower the body, then push through the arms to lift back up. Do not push up using the gluteals – you should feel this in the back of the arms.

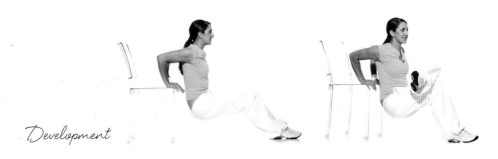

Development

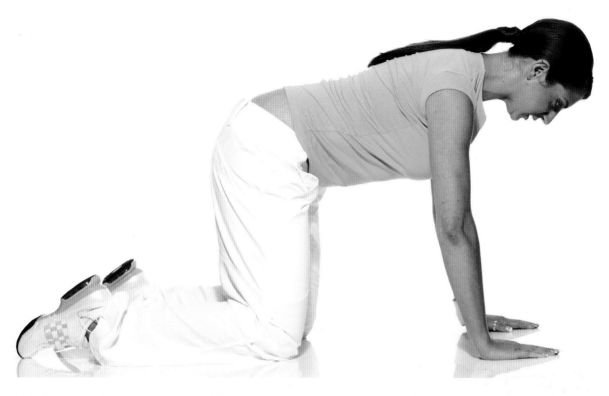

Abdominal Contractions on All Fours

Get on all fours so you are in a table-top position (back flat, hands underneath the shoulders and knees underneath the hips). Breathe in wide into the ribcage. Breathe out and draw the navel to the spine without moving the back. Breathe in and hold this position. Breathe out and release the abdominal contraction without moving the back.

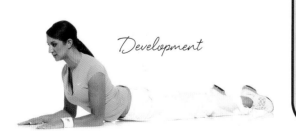

Development

SETS: 1
REPS LEVEL 1: 10
     LEVEL 2: 10
     LEVEL 3: 10
DEVELOPMENT:
- Lie on your front with bent elbows underneath the shoulders (sphinx position). Your pelvis may begin to leave the floor.

MUSCLES WORKED: abdominals

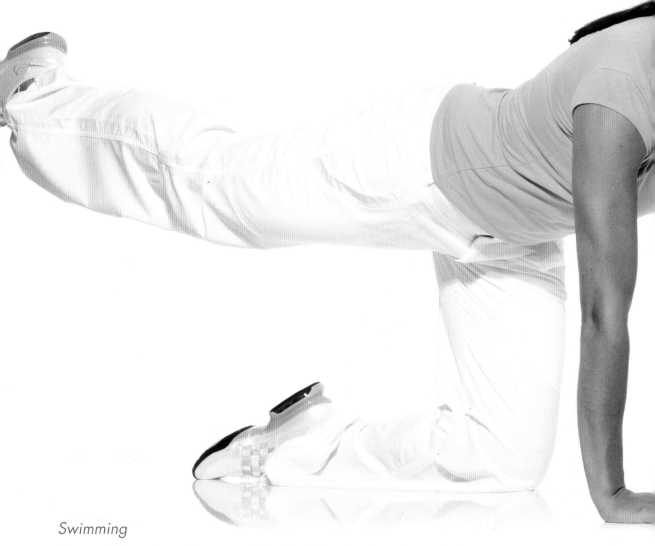

Swimming

Get on all fours in a table-top position (back flat, hands underneath the shoulders and knees underneath the hips). Draw the navel to the spine (as before) to prepare. Breathe in, then breathe out as you lengthen and extend opposite arm and leg, maintaining a flat back and without dipping or lifting the shoulders or hips (keep the weight central and don't transfer all the weight onto one side of hip). Breathe in to return smoothly to the starting position. Do once on each side.

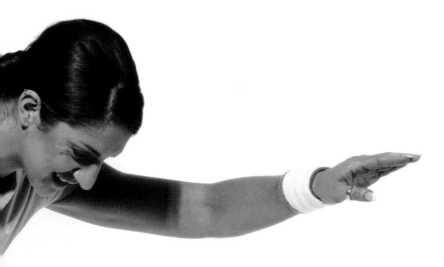

SETS: 1 (each side)

STRETCH TO RELEASE: sit back on your heels with the head on the floor and the arms in front of you – feel the back lengthen.

REPS LEVEL 1: 8

    LEVEL 2: 10

    LEVEL 3: 12

DEVELOPMENT:

- Start with the hand and opposite knee lifted 2 centimetres from the floor, extend your arm and leg and return to hover.
- Lie on your front with bent elbows underneath the shoulders. Push up to half plank position. Extend opposite arm and leg. Breathe in to return to starting position. Repeat on other side.
- Start with the hands under the shoulders and lift the knees to balance on toes. Extend opposite arm and leg. Breathe in to return to starting position. Repeat on one side until set is complete. Perform stretches on pages 84–7. Repeat on other side.

MUSCLES WORKED: abdominals, gluteals

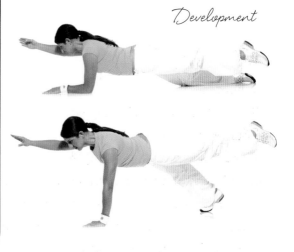

Development

Abdominal Crunch

Lie flat on your back with your legs and feet slightly wider than your hips. Place your hands behind the head to support it. On no account pull on the head. Breathe out and draw the abdominals in, navel to spine, and curl the upper body up off the floor. Aim to draw the ribcage down towards the hips so that the abdominal wall contracts flat and compact – don't let the abdominals dome. Keep a small gap between the chin and the chest. Breathe in to lower yourself back to the starting position. The slower you do this the more effectively your muscles work.

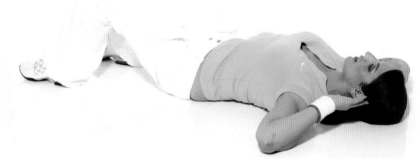

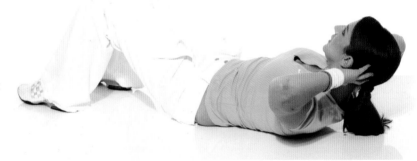

Development

SETS: 2

STRETCH TO RELEASE: sit back on your heels with the head on the floor and the arms in front of you – feel the back lengthen.

REPS LEVEL 1: 10–12

LEVEL 2: 12–15

LEVEL 3: 15–20

DEVELOPMENT:

- As you curl up lift one leg up to 90° from the floor then swap legs halfway through.
- Lift both legs before you curl.

MUSCLES WORKED: abdominals

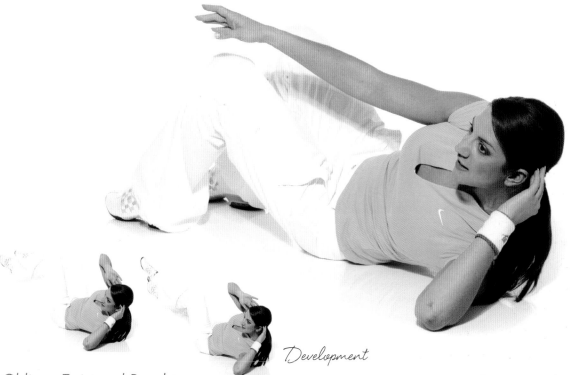

Development

Oblique Twist and Reach

Lie flat on your back with your legs and
feet slightly wider than your hips. Place one
hand behind the head to support it. Do not
pull on the head. Breathe out and draw the
abdominals in, navel to spine, and lift the
upper body. Aim to draw the ribcage down
towards the hips so that the abdominal wall
contracts flat and compact – don't let the
abdominals dome – keep a small gap between
the chin and the chest. Reach the free arm
over to the opposite knee, aiming to take the
shoulder away from the floor as you twist
across the body. Breathe in to lower. Repeat
on the other side.

Finish with the stretches on pages 84–7.

SETS: 1 (on each side)
STRETCH TO RELEASE: sit back on your heels
with the head on the floor and the arms in
front of you – feel the back lengthen.
REPS LEVEL 1: 10–12
     LEVEL 2: 12–15
     LEVEL 3: 15–20
DEVELOPMENT:
- Start with both legs lifted and aim to twist
the shoulder to the knee – do not cheat by
bringing the knees towards the shoulder.
- Start with both legs lifted and aim to twist
the shoulder to the knee, extending the
opposite leg at the same time.
MUSCLES WORKED: abdominals-obliques

WORKOUT THREE
SPLIT SESSIONS – CHEST AND ARMS

Workouts three, four and five all target specific areas of the body but also include core exercises to improve your abdominals and back muscles, which are essential for good posture and strength.

Hand weights are used for many of these exercises and you can make them at home by using two water–filled bottles or, to make them heavier, fill an empty bottle with sugar to the required weight.

Warm-up: 5 minutes stretching/mobility (see pages 84–7 and 96–7); 10–20 minutes cardiovascular activity (see pages 106–111)

Press-Ups

Start on all fours, have your hands wider than your shoulders, fingers pointing forwards. Engage your abdominals and lower the chest to the floor, bending the elbows, as you breathe in. Breathe out, engage the abdominals as you push the hands into the floor to lift the body back up. A full press-up is one with the legs stretched out behind you and toes tucked underneath (for illustration, see page 124).

SETS: 2
REST PERIOD BETWEEN SETS:
    30–60 seconds
REPS LEVEL 1: 10–12
        LEVEL 2: 12–15
        LEVEL 3: 15–20
DEVELOPMENT:
• Full press-up.
MUSCLES WORKED:
    abdominals, chest, triceps

SETS: 2

REST PERIOD BETWEEN SETS:
   30–60 seconds

REPS LEVEL 1: 10–12

      LEVEL 2: 12–15

      LEVEL 3: 15–20

DEVELOPMENT:
- Increase the weight.
- Stand on one leg.

MUSCLES WORKED: biceps

Biceps Curl

Stand with your feet shoulder-distance apart, with a weight in each hand and your arms by your sides. Your hands should face forward. Keeping the elbows in to the sides bend them and lift the weights. Do not swing the trunk as you lift. Lower the arms back to the sides. Keep the elbows soft.

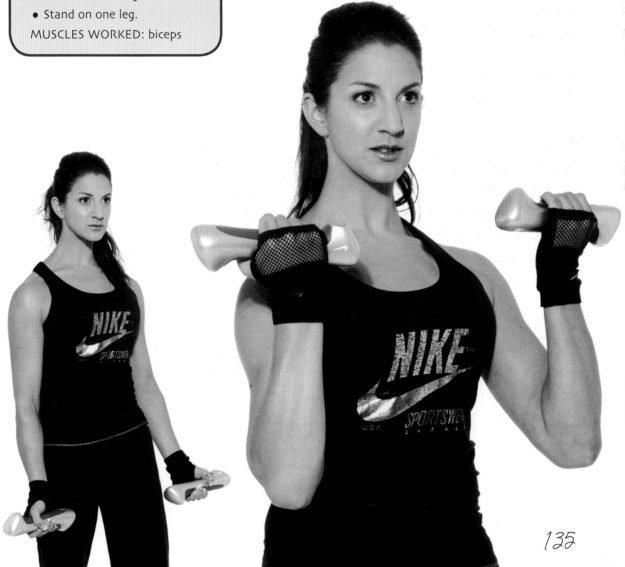

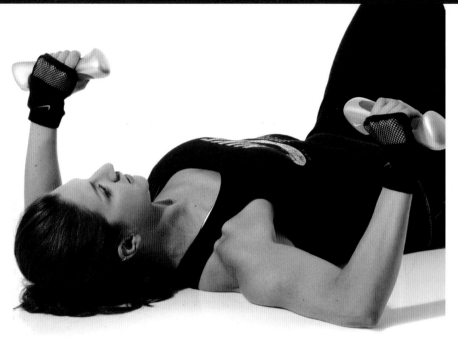

Chest Press

Lie on your back on the floor with the knees bent and feet flat on the floor and parallel with the hips. Hold a weight in each hand. Have the elbows on the floor at chest level, with the palms facing forwards, knuckles pointing towards the ceiling. Keeping the elbows in line with the wrists, push both hands up and extend the arms over the centre of the chest, lower them back down, and lightly touch the elbows to the floor before the next repetition.

SETS: 2
REST PERIOD BETWEEN SETS: 15–30 seconds
REPS LEVEL 1: 10–12
      LEVEL 2: 12–15
      LEVEL 3: 15–20
DEVELOPMENT:
• Increase the weight.
MUSCLES WORKED: chest, biceps

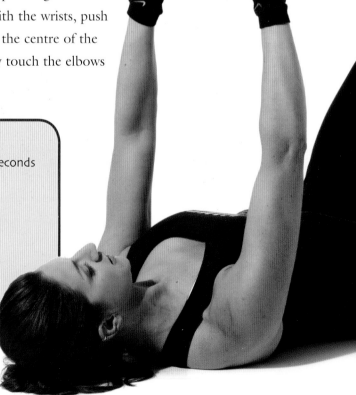

Triceps Dips

Place a chair against a wall and sit on it
with your knees bent and feet hip-distance
apart. Have your hands on the edge of the
chair with the fingers pointing forward.
Straighten the arms to lift the bottom
up away from the chair. Bend the elbows
directly behind you to lower the body,
then push through the arms to lift back up.
Do not push up using the gluteals – you
should feel this in the back of the arms
(for illustration see page 128).

> SETS: 2
> REST PERIOD BETWEEN SETS: 30–60 seconds
> REPS LEVEL 1: 10–12
> LEVEL 2: 12–15
> LEVEL 3: 15–20
> DEVELOPMENT:
> - Take the legs further away
>   or straighten.
> - Cross one leg over the other.
> - Change position halfway through.
> MUSCLES WORKED: triceps

Abdominal Contractions on All Fours

Get on all fours so you are in a table-top
position (back flat, hands underneath the
shoulders and knees underneath the hips).
Breathe in wide into the ribcage. Breathe
out and draw the navel to the spine
without moving the back. Breathe in and
hold this position. Breathe out and release
the contraction without moving the back
(for illustration see page 129).

> SETS: 1
> REPS LEVEL 1: 10
> LEVEL 2: 10
> LEVEL 3: 10
> DEVELOPMENT:
> - Lie on your front with bent elbows
>   underneath the shoulders (sphinx position).
>   Your pelvis may begin to leave the floor.
> MUSCLES WORKED: abdominals

SETS: 2
REST PERIOD BETWEEN SETS:
    30–60 seconds
REPS LEVEL 1: 15–20
        LEVEL 2: 20–30
        LEVEL 3: 30–50
DEVELOPMENT:
- Increase the weight.
- Perform from a shoulder bridge position (feet on the floor, lift the hips so you come up onto your shoulder blades).
MUSCLES WORKED: chest

Chest Flies

Lie on your back with a weight in each hand and your arms stretched above the chest, elbows soft and palms facing. Lower the weights sideways to shoulder level and return back to the starting position – do NOT arch the back as you lower and lift, keep the abdominals engaged.

SETS: 2

REST PERIOD BETWEEN SETS: 30–60 seconds

REPS LEVEL 1: 8–10 each phase

      LEVEL 2: 10–12 each phase

      LEVEL 3: 12–15 each phase

DEVELOPMENT:

- Increase weight.
- Perform standing on one leg.

MUSCLES WORKED: biceps

Biceps Combo

Stand with your feet shoulder-distance apart. Hold a weight in each hand, arms down by your sides and palms facing forward.

Phase 1: bend the elbows so they are at right angles. Keep the elbows in to the sides. Do not swing the trunk as you lift. Lower the arms. Keep the elbows soft.

Phase 2: Lift the weights so the elbows are at a right angle, pause, then from here lift to the top and back down to halfway.

Phase 3: Lift all the way up to the shoulder and all the way down.

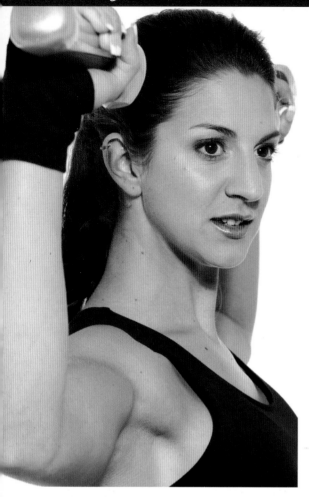

Seated Pec Dec

Sit on a chair with the back supported. Have a weight in each hand at shoulder height, and the elbows at right angles. Squeeze the arms together keeping the wrists and elbows in line and then open to return to the starting position.

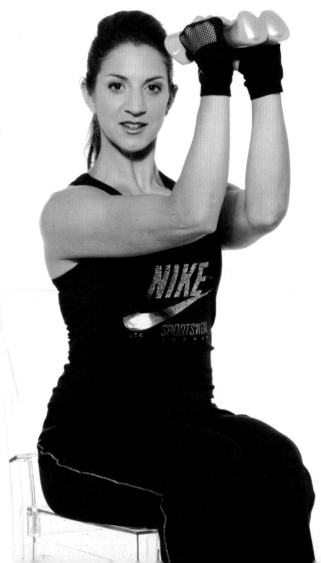

SETS: 2
REPS LEVEL 1: 10–12
LEVEL 2: 12–15
LEVEL 3: 15–20
DEVELOPMENT:
- Increase weight.
- Perform standing.
MUSCLES WORKED: chest

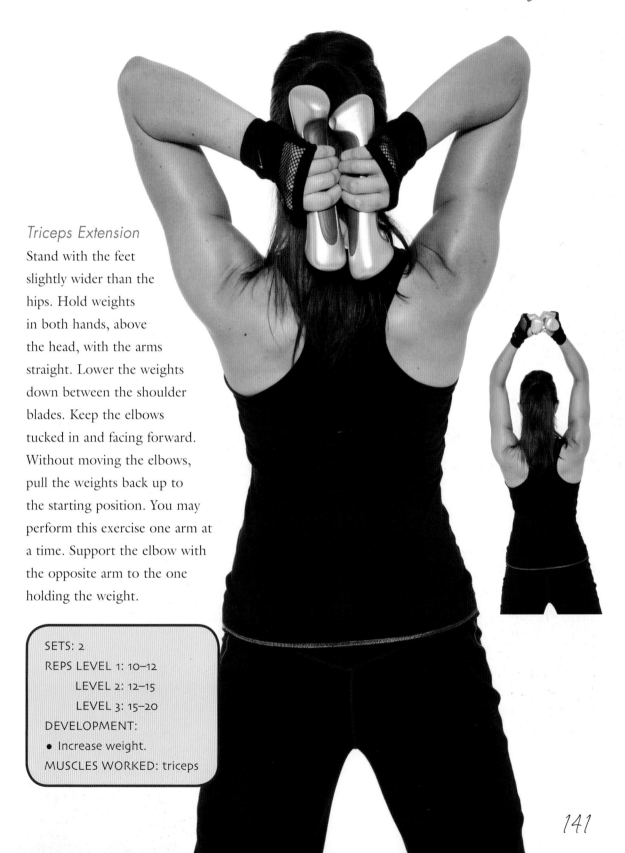

Triceps Extension

Stand with the feet slightly wider than the hips. Hold weights in both hands, above the head, with the arms straight. Lower the weights down between the shoulder blades. Keep the elbows tucked in and facing forward. Without moving the elbows, pull the weights back up to the starting position. You may perform this exercise one arm at a time. Support the elbow with the opposite arm to the one holding the weight.

SETS: 2
REPS LEVEL 1: 10–12
LEVEL 2: 12–15
LEVEL 3: 15–20
DEVELOPMENT:
• Increase weight.
MUSCLES WORKED: triceps

Oblique Twist and Reach

Lie flat on your back with your legs and feet slightly wider than your hips. Place one hand behind the head to support it. Do not pull on the head. Breathe out and draw the abdominals in, navel to spine, and lift the upper body. Aim to draw the ribcage down towards the hips so that the abdominal wall contracts flat and compact – don't let the abdominals dome and keep a small gap between the chin and the chest. Reach the free arm over to the opposite knee, aiming to take the shoulder away from the floor as you twist across the body. Breathe in to lower. Repeat on the other side (for illustration see page 133).

SETS: 1 (one on each side)

STRETCH TO RELEASE: sit back on your heels with the head on the floor and the arms in front of you – feel the back lengthen.

REPS LEVEL 1: 10–12

   LEVEL 2: 12–15

   LEVEL 3: 15–20

DEVELOPMENT:

- Start with both legs lifted and aim to twist the shoulder to the knee – do not cheat by bringing the knees towards the shoulder.
- Start with both legs lifted and aim to twist shoulder to knee, extending the opposite leg at the same time.

MUSCLES WORKED: abdominals-obliques

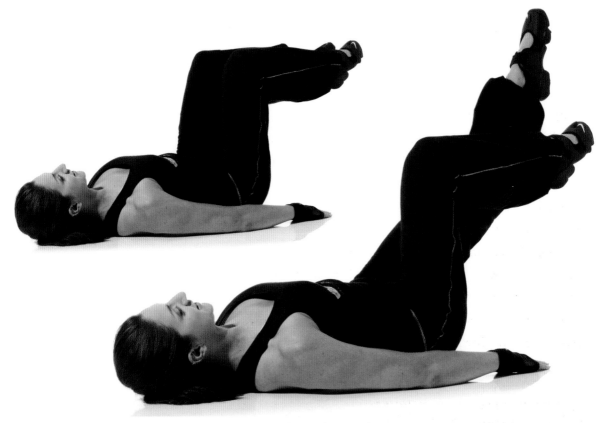

Leg Extensions

Lie on the back with the knees
bent at right angles above the
hips. Breathe in to prepare.
Breathe out, draw navel to spine
as you extend one leg away from
you – do NOT allow the back to
arch or the abdominals to dome.
Breathe in as you return the foot
back to its starting position, then
repeat on the opposite side.

SETS: 2

STRETCH TO RELEASE: sit back on your heels with the
head on the floor and the arms in front of you – feel
the back lengthen.

REPS LEVEL 1: 10–15 (one leg at a time)

LEVEL 2: 10–15 (one or both legs at the same time)

LEVEL 3: 10–15 (both legs)

DEVELOPMENT:

- Start with the knees over the hips, shins parallel to the
floor, extend one leg and, as you bend the knee back
over the hip, extend the other leg.
- Extend both legs together then retract maintaining a
strong, stable back – don't let it arch.
- To challenge your abdominal strength, lower the legs
closer to the floor.

MUSCLES WORKED: abdominals

Plank

Lie on your tummy propped up on your elbows, which should be directly underneath your shoulders. Draw the shoulders back and down towards the waist.

- **Level 1:** draw navel to spine and peel the pelvis away from the floor. Hold and maintain regular breathing.
- **Level 2:** draw navel to spine and lift further so that the bottom is level with the spine but the weight is still distributed between knees and elbows. Hold and maintain regular breathing.
- **Level 3:** draw navel to spine, lift the pelvis and knees off the floor, keep the spine level and lengthened. Hold and maintain regular breathing.

Finish with the stretches on pages 86–7.

SETS: 3

STRETCH TO RELEASE: sit back on your heels with the head on the floor and the arms in front of you – feel the back lengthen.

REPS LEVEL 1: 20–30 seconds

LEVEL 2: 30–45 seconds

LEVEL 3: 45 seconds–1 minute

DEVELOPMENT:

- Do a half plank and lift one leg.
- Do a full plank and lift one leg.

MUSCLES WORKED: abdominals

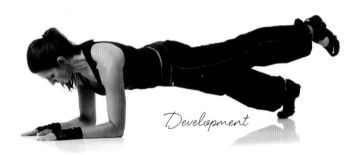

Development

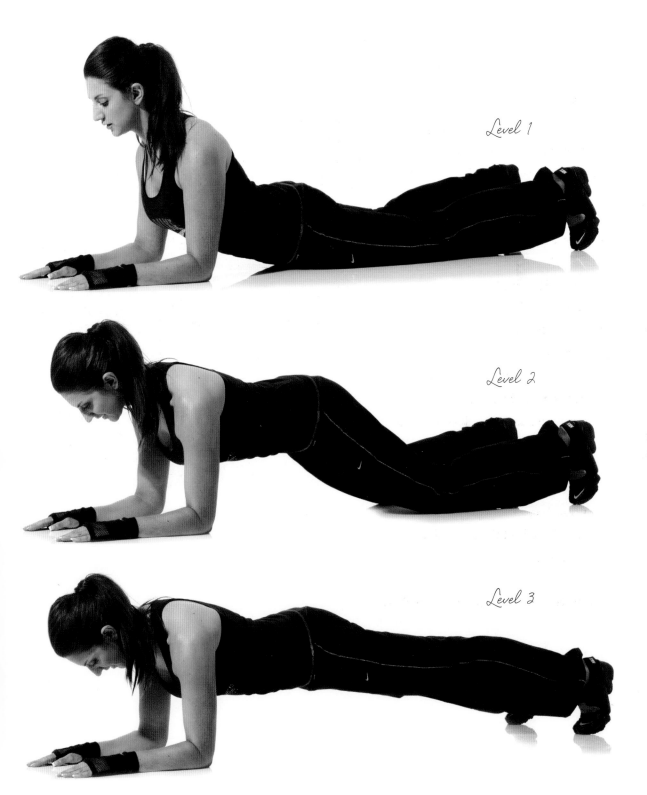

Level 1

Level 2

Level 3

WORKOUT FOUR
SPLIT SESSIONS – BACK AND SHOULDERS

Hand weights are used for many of these exercises and you can make them at home by using two water–filled bottles or, to make them heavier, fill an empty bottle with sugar to the required weight.

Warm-up: 5 minutes stretching/mobility (see pages 84–7 and 96–7); 10–20 minutes cardiovascular activity (see pages 106–111)

Weighted Shoulder Press

Stand with the feet hip-width apart and with a weight in each hand, arms at shoulder height. Keep elbows underneath the wrists. Push up above the head but slightly in front (so you can see your hands at all times), don't lock the elbows. Return to the starting position (for illustration see page 125).

> SETS: 2
> REST PERIOD BETWEEN SETS:
>   30–60 seconds
> REPS LEVEL 1: 10–12
>   LEVEL 2: 12–15
>   LEVEL 3: 15–20
> DEVELOPMENT:
> • Increase the weight.
> • Perform standing on one leg.
> MUSCLES WORKED: shoulders

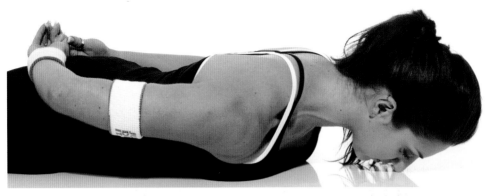

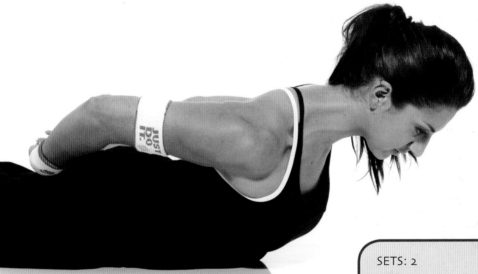

Back Extension

Lie on your tummy. Connect navel to spine to engage the abdominals. Extend and lengthen through the spine so that the upper back slightly lifts from the floor, then lower down with control. Don't over-arch the back.

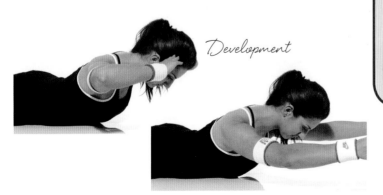

Development

SETS: 2

REST PERIOD BETWEEN SETS:
　30–60 seconds

REPS LEVEL 1: 10–12

　　　LEVEL 2: 12–15

　　　LEVEL 3: 15–20

DEVELOPMENT:

● Bend the elbows and place the fingertips on the head.

● Extend the arms in front.

MUSCLES WORKED: back, abdominals

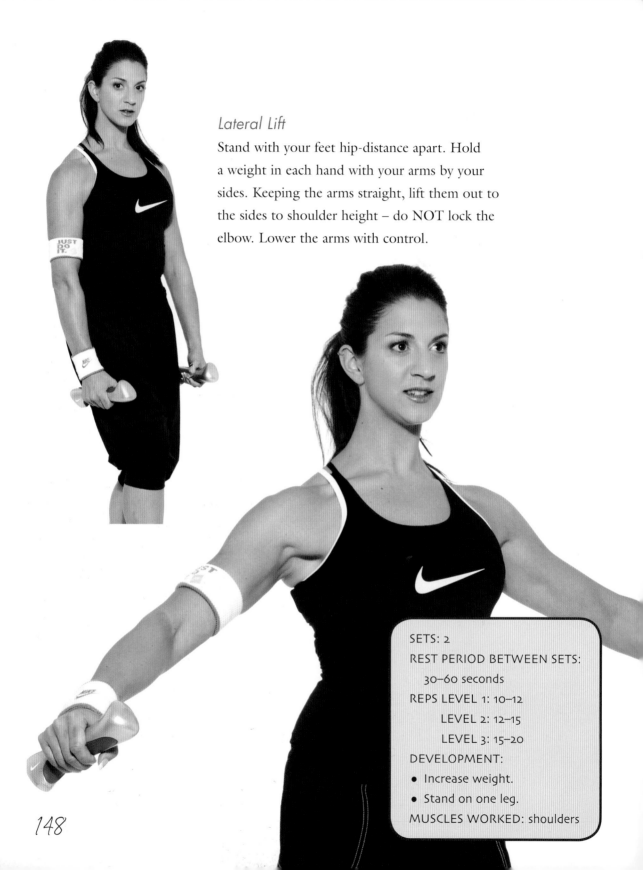

Lateral Lift

Stand with your feet hip-distance apart. Hold a weight in each hand with your arms by your sides. Keeping the arms straight, lift them out to the sides to shoulder height – do NOT lock the elbow. Lower the arms with control.

SETS: 2

REST PERIOD BETWEEN SETS:
   30–60 seconds

REPS LEVEL 1: 10–12

   LEVEL 2: 12–15

   LEVEL 3: 15–20

DEVELOPMENT:

- Increase weight.
- Stand on one leg.

MUSCLES WORKED: shoulders

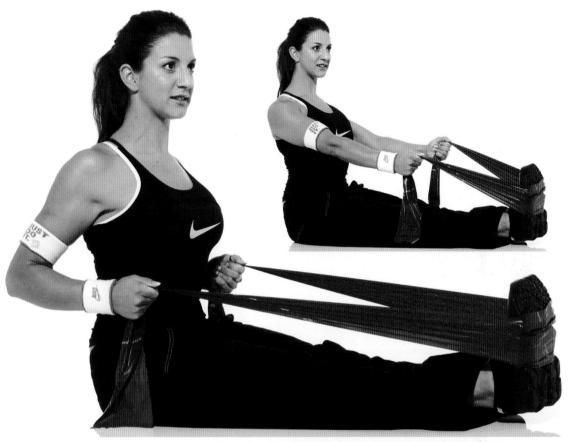

Cable Row

Sit up straight with your legs extended and knees slightly bent. Put a band around the soles of the feet. Tuck the elbows in to the sides and draw them back so you can feel the shoulder blades nipping together. Lengthen the arms back to the starting position.

If you don't have a band, bend forwards from hips with a weight in each hand and your arms lengthening forward, then pull the arms upwards and towards the sides, nipping the shoulder blades together. Relax the arms.

SETS: 2
REST PERIOD BETWEEN SETS: 30–60 seconds
REPS LEVEL 1: 10–12
      LEVEL 2: 12–15
      LEVEL 3: 15–20
DEVELOPMENT:
● Make the movement slow.
MUSCLES WORKED: latissimus dorsi

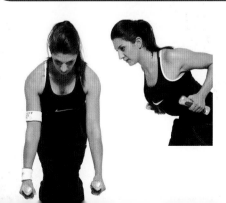

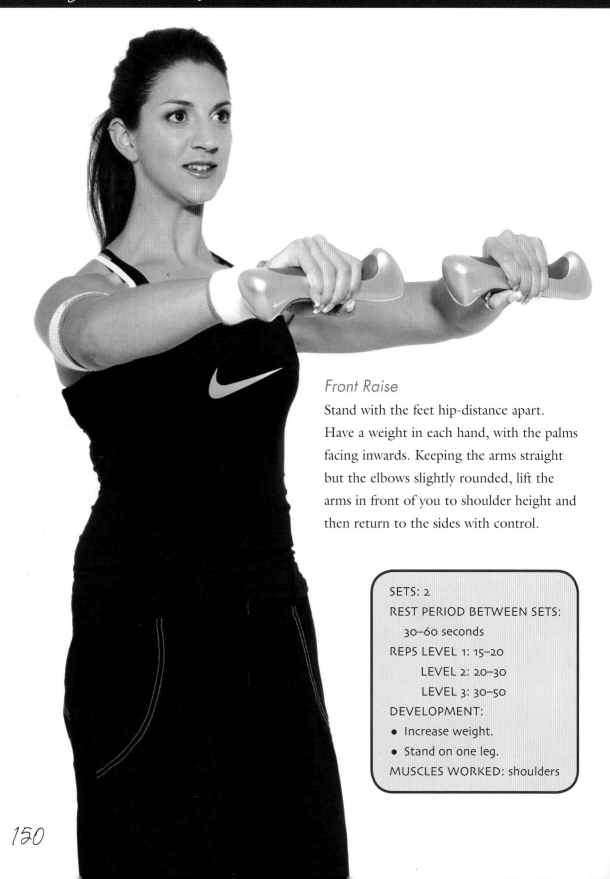

Front Raise

Stand with the feet hip-distance apart.
Have a weight in each hand, with the palms
facing inwards. Keeping the arms straight
but the elbows slightly rounded, lift the
arms in front of you to shoulder height and
then return to the sides with control.

SETS: 2
REST PERIOD BETWEEN SETS:
  30–60 seconds
REPS LEVEL 1: 15–20
       LEVEL 2: 20–30
       LEVEL 3: 30–50
DEVELOPMENT:
• Increase weight.
• Stand on one leg.
MUSCLES WORKED: shoulders

Swimming

Get on all fours in a table-top
position (back flat, hands underneath
the shoulders and knees underneath
the hips). Draw the navel to the
spine to prepare. Breathe in, then
breathe out as you lengthen and
extend opposite arm and leg,
maintaining a flat back and without
dipping or lifting the shoulders
or hips (keep the weight central
and don't transfer all the weight
onto one side of hip). Breathe in
to return smoothly to the starting
position. Do once on each side (for
illustration see pages 130–31).

SETS: 1 (one on each side)
STRETCH TO RELEASE: Sit back on your heels with
    the head on the floor and the arms in front of you
    – feel the back lengthen.
REPS LEVEL 1: 8
    LEVEL 2: 10
    LEVEL 3: 12
DEVELOPMENT:
- Start with the hand and opposite knee lifted 2
  centimetres from the floor, extend your arm and
  leg and return to hover.
- Lie on your front with bent elbows underneath the
  shoulders. Push up to half plank position. Extend
  opposite arm and leg. Breathe in to return to
  starting position. Repeat on other side.
- Start with the hands under the shoulders and lift
  the knees to balance on toes. Extend opposite arm
  and leg. Breathe in to return to starting position.
  Repeat on one side until set is complete. Perform
  stretches on pages 92–5. Repeat on other side.
MUSCLES WORKED: abdominals, gluteals

SETS: 2
REST PERIOD BETWEEN SETS: 30–60 seconds
REPS LEVEL 1: 10
    LEVEL 2: 10
    LEVEL 3: 10
DEVELOPMENT:
- Lie on your front with bent elbows
  underneath the shoulders (sphinx position).
  Your pelvis may begin to leave the floor.
MUSCLES WORKED: abdominals

Abdominal Contractions on All Fours

Get on all fours so you are in a table-top
position (back flat, hands underneath the
shoulders and knees underneath the hips).
Breathe in wide into the ribcage. Breathe
out and draw the navel to the spine without
moving the back. Breathe in and hold
this position. Breathe out and release the
contraction without moving the back (for
illustration see page 129).

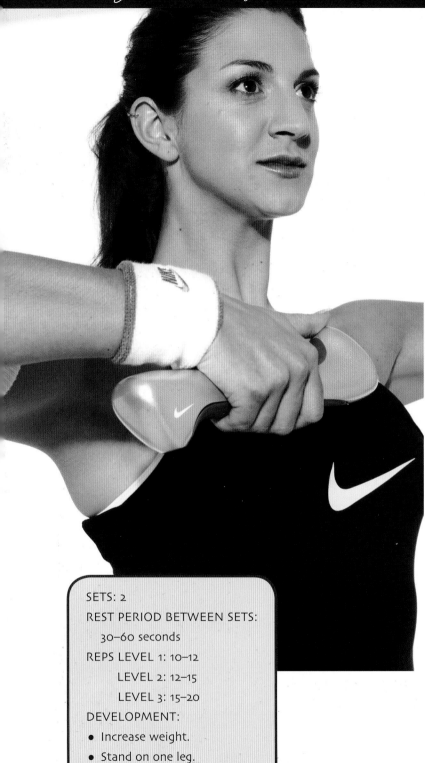

Upright Row

Stand with the feet slightly wider than the hips. Hold a weight in each hand in front of each thigh with your palms towards you. Breathe out and bend the elbows to lift the weights up to the chest – do not swing the trunk, and make sure your wrists stay in line with your forearms. Breathe in and lower; don't lock the elbows.

SETS: 2
REST PERIOD BETWEEN SETS:
   30–60 seconds
REPS LEVEL 1: 10–12
     LEVEL 2: 12–15
     LEVEL 3: 15–20
DEVELOPMENT:
• Increase weight.
• Stand on one leg.
MUSCLES WORKED: shoulders

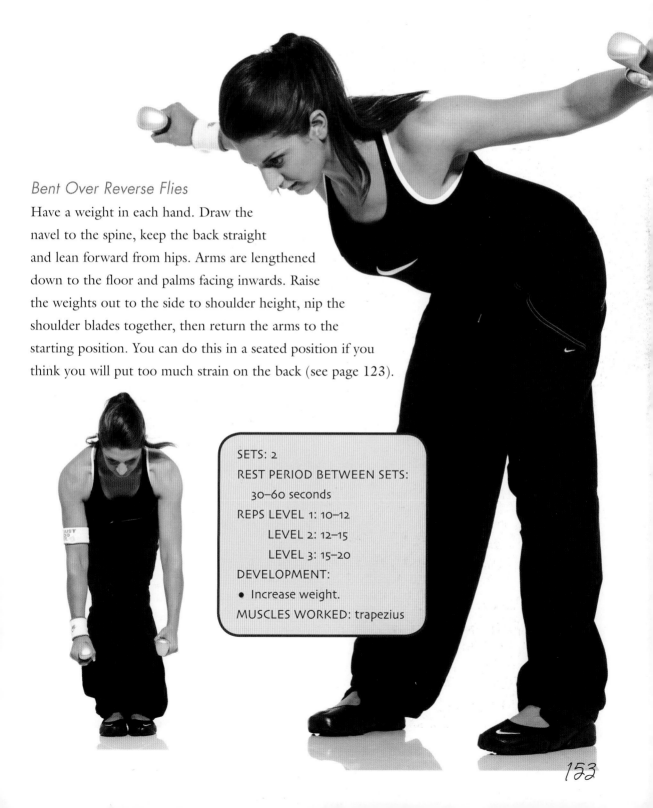

Bent Over Reverse Flies

Have a weight in each hand. Draw the
navel to the spine, keep the back straight
and lean forward from hips. Arms are lengthened
down to the floor and palms facing inwards. Raise
the weights out to the side to shoulder height, nip the
shoulder blades together, then return the arms to the
starting position. You can do this in a seated position if you
think you will put too much strain on the back (see page 123).

SETS: 2
REST PERIOD BETWEEN SETS:
   30–60 seconds
REPS LEVEL 1: 10–12
         LEVEL 2: 12–15
         LEVEL 3: 15–20
DEVELOPMENT:
● Increase weight.
MUSCLES WORKED: trapezius

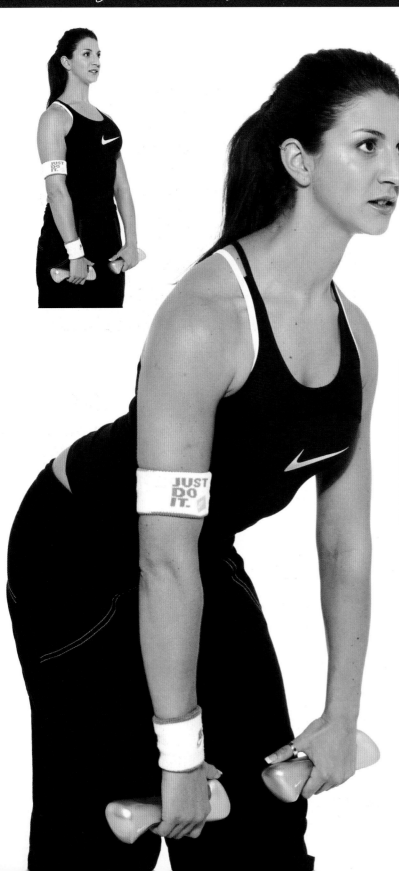

SETS: 2
REST PERIOD BETWEEN SETS:
  30–60 seconds
REPS LEVEL 1: 10–12
    LEVEL 2: 12–15
    LEVEL 3: 15–20
DEVELOPMENT:
• Increase weight.
MUSCLES WORKED: back

Deadlift

Stand with your feet slightly wider
than the hips. Hold a medium to
heavy weight (between 3 and 8
kilos) in each hand. Contract your
abdominals and, keeping the knees
slightly bent and the back straight,
slowly hinge forward from the
hips. Keep your hands close to
your thighs. Straighten up.

Plank

Lie on your tummy propped up on your elbows, which should be directly underneath your shoulders. Draw the shoulders back and down towards the waist.

- **Level 1:** draw navel to spine and peel the pelvis away from the floor. Hold and maintain regular breathing.

- **Level 2:** draw navel to spine and lift further so that the bottom is level with the spine but the weight is still distributed between knees and elbows. Hold and maintain regular breathing.

- **Level 3:** draw navel to spine, lift the pelvis and knees off the floor, keep the spine level and lengthened. Hold and maintain regular breathing.

SETS: 3

STRETCH TO RELEASE: sit back on your heels with the head on the floor and the arms in front of you – feel the back lengthen

REPS LEVEL 1: 20–30 seconds

   LEVEL 2: 30–45 seconds

   LEVEL 3: 45 seconds–1 minute

DEVELOPMENT:

- Do a half plank and lift one leg.
- Do a full plank and lift one leg.

MUSCLES WORKED: abdominals

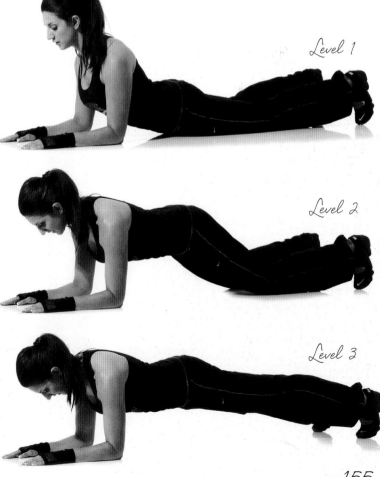

Level 1

Level 2

Level 3

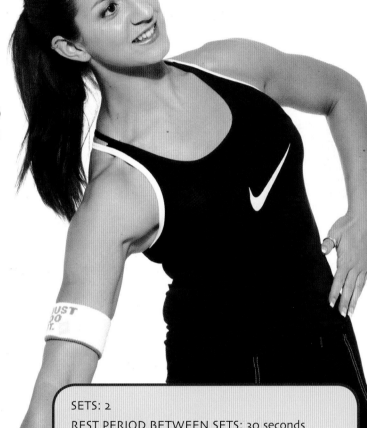

Side Bends

Stand with the feet slightly wider than the hips. Hold a medium to heavy weight (between 3 and 8 kilos) in one hand and have the other hand on the hip. Pull in the abdominals as you reach over sideways, then use the muscles in your side to pull yourself back to standing upright – do NOT throw the hips to the side, keep them centred. Repeat on the opposite side.

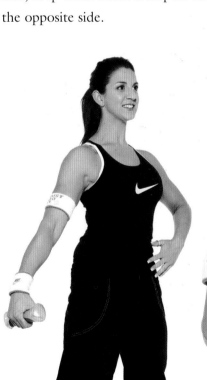

SETS: 2

REST PERIOD BETWEEN SETS: 30 seconds

REPS LEVEL 1: 10–15 (alternating sides)

LEVEL 2: 10–15 (once or twice on each side)

LEVEL 3: 10–15 (twice on each side)

DEVELOPMENT:

• Increase weight.

MUSCLES WORKED: abdominals-obliques

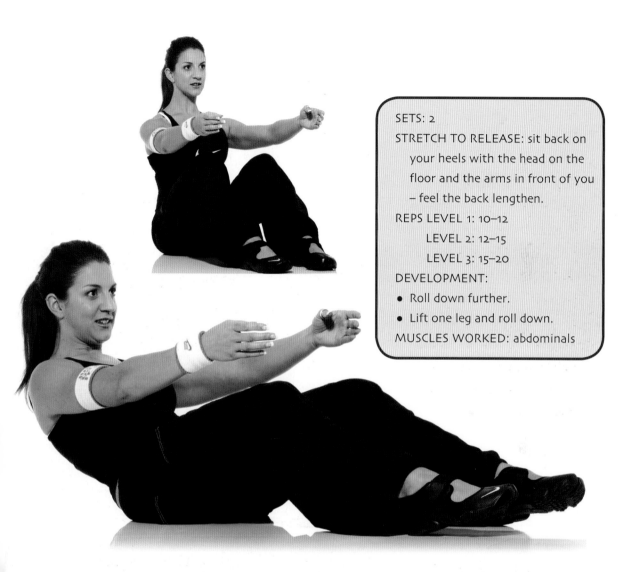

SETS: 2

STRETCH TO RELEASE: sit back on your heels with the head on the floor and the arms in front of you – feel the back lengthen.

REPS LEVEL 1: 10–12

LEVEL 2: 12–15

LEVEL 3: 15–20

DEVELOPMENT:

- Roll down further.
- Lift one leg and roll down.

MUSCLES WORKED: abdominals

Reverse Sit Up (Roll Down)

Sit upright on your sitting bones (right at the bottom of your pelvis). You can have your knees bent or legs straight in front of you. Keep the legs together. Pull in your abdominals and tuck the pelvis underneath you as you roll slowly down towards the floor to a position where you feel your abdominals contract effectively without any doming. Keep your back curved as you go down and as you come up.

Finish with the stretches on pages 84–7.

WORKOUT FIVE
SPLIT SESSIONS – LEGS

Hand weights are used for many of these exercises and you can make them at home by using two water–filled bottles or, to make them heavier, fill an empty bottle with sugar to the required weight.

Warm-up: 5 minutes stretching/mobility (see pages 84–7 and 96–7); 10–20 minutes cardiovascular activity (see pages 106–111)

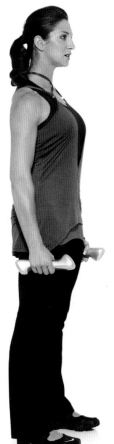

Weighted Squats

Hold a weight in each hand and stand with the feet slightly wider than the hips. The feet should be parallel and the toes pointing forward. Keep the weight in the heels and think of the chest lifting as you bend the knees. Send the tailbone (the last bone in your spine) backwards while maintaining a flat back. Breathe out as you return to standing, slightly squeezing the abdominals and gluteals as you lift the body.

SETS: 2
REST PERIOD BETWEEN SETS:
  30–60 seconds
REPS LEVEL 1: 10–12
       LEVEL 2: 12–15
       LEVEL 3: 15–20
DEVELOPMENT:
• Increase weight.
• Stand on one leg.
MUSCLES WORKED: quads,
  hamstrings, gluteals

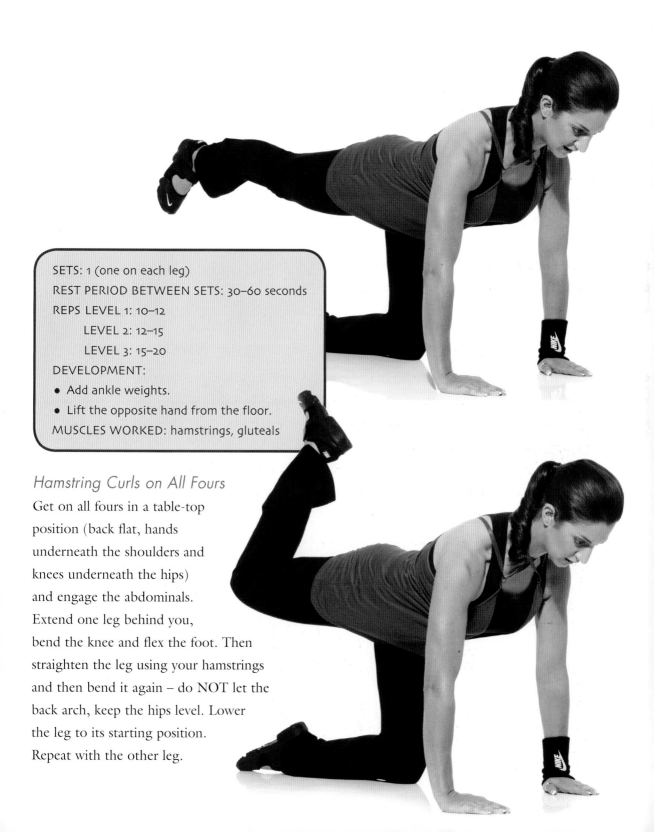

SETS: 1 (one on each leg)

REST PERIOD BETWEEN SETS: 30–60 seconds

REPS LEVEL 1: 10–12

LEVEL 2: 12–15

LEVEL 3: 15–20

DEVELOPMENT:

- Add ankle weights.
- Lift the opposite hand from the floor.

MUSCLES WORKED: hamstrings, gluteals

Hamstring Curls on All Fours

Get on all fours in a table-top
position (back flat, hands
underneath the shoulders and
knees underneath the hips)
and engage the abdominals.
Extend one leg behind you,
bend the knee and flex the foot. Then
straighten the leg using your hamstrings
and then bend it again – do NOT let the
back arch, keep the hips level. Lower
the leg to its starting position.
Repeat with the other leg.

SETS: 2
REST PERIOD BETWEEN SETS: 30–60 seconds
REPS LEVEL 1: 10–12
      LEVEL 2: 12–15
      LEVEL 3: 15–20
DEVELOPMENT:
- Make the lunges a non–stop pulsing action.
- Don't come all the way to the top before lowering back down.

MUSCLES WORKED: quads, hamstrings, gluteals

Lunges

Stand with feet hip-width apart, with one foot forward and one back. Lift the heel of the back foot. Lower body down (not forwards) until you adopt a right angle with the back knee (your front knee should bend so your knee is above the ankle – NOT over the toe). Straighten back to the starting position (for illustration see page 126).

Abdominal Contractions on All Fours

Get on all fours so you are in a table-top position (back flat, hands underneath the shoulders and knees underneath the hips). Breathe in wide into the ribcage. Breathe out and draw the navel to the spine without moving the back. Breathe in and hold this position. Breathe out and release the contraction without moving the back (for illustration see page 129).

SETS: 1
REPS LEVEL 1: 10
      LEVEL 2: 10
      LEVEL 3: 10
DEVELOPMENT:
- Lie on your front with bent elbows underneath the shoulders (sphinx position). Your pelvis may begin to leave the floor.

MUSCLES WORKED: abdominals

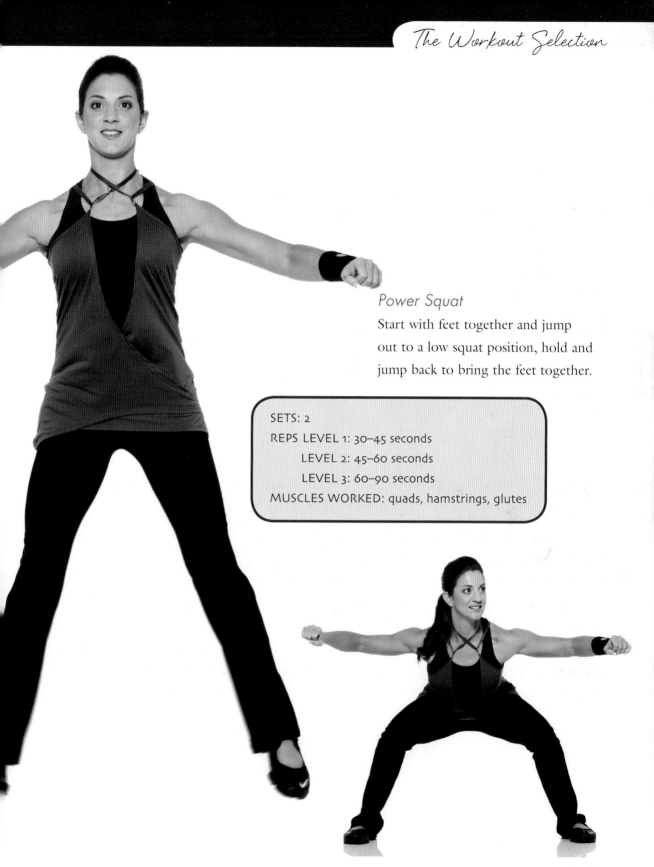

Power Squat

Start with feet together and jump
out to a low squat position, hold and
jump back to bring the feet together.

SETS: 2
REPS LEVEL 1: 30–45 seconds
      LEVEL 2: 45–60 seconds
      LEVEL 3: 60–90 seconds
MUSCLES WORKED: quads, hamstrings, glutes

Glute Squeezes on All Fours

Get on all fours in a table-top position (back flat, hands underneath the shoulders and knees underneath the hips) and engage the abdominals. Lower the forearms to rest on the floor. Extend one leg behind you, bend the knee and flex the foot. Squeeze the glutes and push up towards the ceiling, focusing on the bottom – do NOT let the back arch, keep the hips level. Lower the leg back to its starting position.

SETS: 2
REST PERIOD BETWEEN SETS:
   30–60 seconds
REPS LEVEL 1: 10–12
        LEVEL 2: 12–15
        LEVEL 3: 15–20
DEVELOPMENT:
● Add ankle weights.
MUSCLES WORKED: gluteals

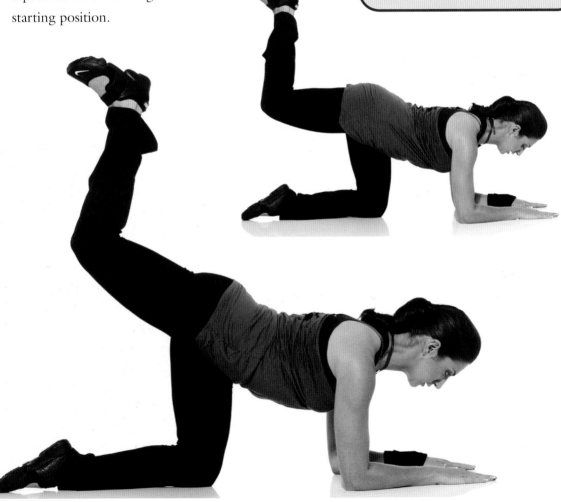

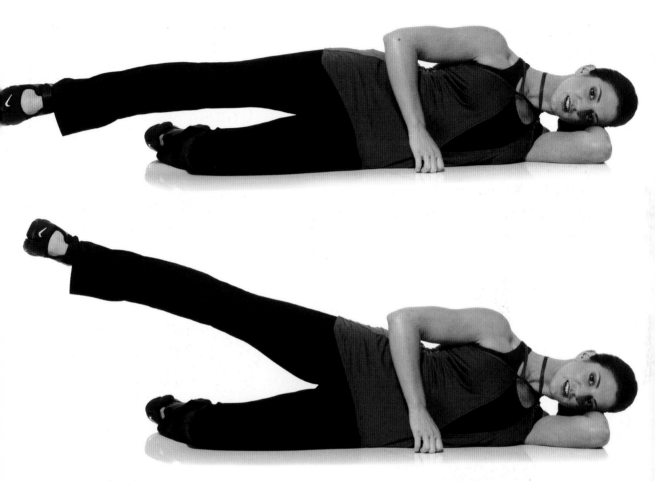

Outer Thigh Lift

Lie on your side with the underneath leg bent slightly forward and the top leg extended. Keep the toes pointing forward as you lift and lower the upper leg. Repeat on the other side.

SETS: 1 (one on each side)
REST PERIOD BETWEEN SETS:
  30–60 seconds
REPS LEVEL 1: 15–20
        LEVEL 2: 20–30
        LEVEL 3: 30–50
DEVELOPMENT:
● Add ankle weights.
MUSCLES WORKED: abductors

Inner Thigh Lift

Lie on your side with the top leg bent slightly forwards, resting the knee on the floor in front of you. Keep the toes pointing forwards as you lift and lower the underneath leg. Repeat on the other side.

SETS: 1 (one on each side)
REST PERIOD BETWEEN SETS:
   30–60 seconds
REPS LEVEL 1: 15–20
      LEVEL 2: 20–30
      LEVEL 3: 30–50
DEVELOPMENT:
- Add ankle weights.
MUSCLES WORKED: adductors

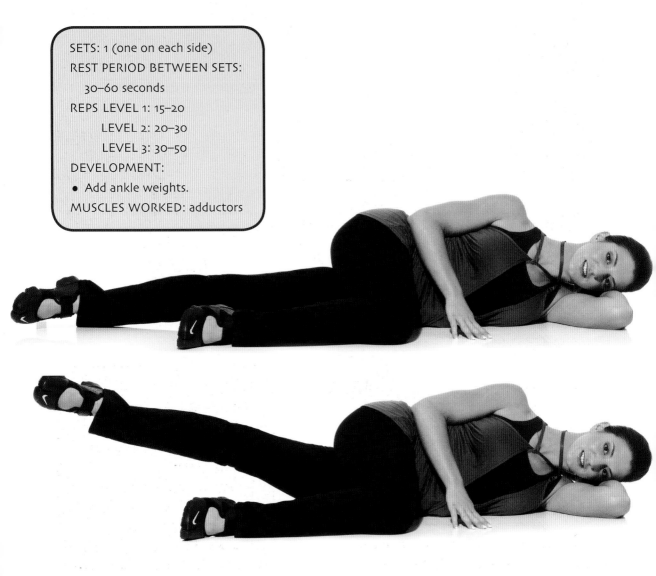

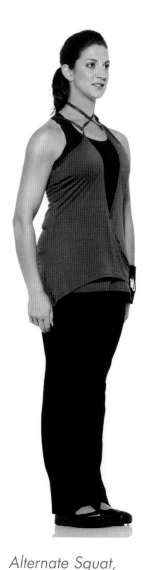

Alternate Squat, Step Out Wide, Step In

Starting with feet together step to one side and squat. Your knees should stay in line with your toes. Keep the weight in the heels and the chest up as you bend, send the tailbone backwards and maintain a flat back. Bring the feet together and repeat on the other side.

SETS: 2
REPS LEVEL 1: 30–45 seconds
LEVEL 2: 45–60 seconds
LEVEL 3: 60–90 seconds
DEVELOPMENT:
- Jump out, squat, jump in (see Power Squat on page 161)
MUSCLES WORKED: quads, hamstrings, gluteals

Double Leg Lift

Lie on your side, shoulders and hips stacked, keep the legs straight, one on top of the other, feet slightly in front of the hips. Pull in the abdominals, squeeze the legs together and lift them off the floor. Lower with control. A set here is just one lift on one side. Do the repetitions on one side first and then your rest period is the time it takes to turn onto the other side to repeat on that side.

SETS: 1
REPS LEVEL 1: 10–12
LEVEL 2: 12–15
LEVEL 3: 15–20
DEVELOPMENT:
● Add ankle weights.
MUSCLES WORKED: abdominals, abductors, adductors

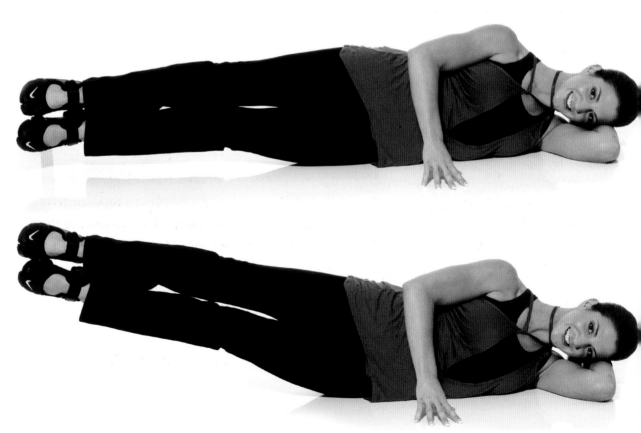

Side Bends

Stand with the feet slightly wider than the hips. Hold a medium to heavy weight (between 3 and 8 kilos) in one hand and have the other hand on the hip. Pull in the abdominals as you reach over sideways, squeeze and pull back to standing – do NOT throw the hips to the side, keep them centred. Repeat on the opposite side (for illustration see page 156).

SETS: 2
REST PERIOD BETWEEN SETS: 30 seconds
REPS LEVEL 1: 10–15 (alternating sides)
        LEVEL 2: 10–15 (once or twice on each side)
        LEVEL 3: 10–15 (twice on each side)
DEVELOPMENT:
• Increase weight.
MUSCLES WORKED: abdominals-obliques

SETS: 2
STRETCH TO RELEASE: sit back on your heels with the head on the floor and the arms in front of you – feel the back lengthen.
REPS LEVEL 1: 10–12
        LEVEL 2: 12–15
        LEVEL 3: 15–20
DEVELOPMENT:
• Roll down further.
• Lift one leg and roll down.
MUSCLES WORKED: abdominals

Reverse Sit Up (Roll Down)

Sit upright on your sitting bones (right at the bottom of your pelvis). You can have your knees bent or legs straight in front of you. Keep the legs together. Pull in your abdominals and tuck the pelvis underneath you as you slowly roll down towards the floor to a position where you feel your abdominals contract effectively without any doming. Keep your back curved as you go down and come up (for illustration see page 157).

Finish with the stretches on pages 84–7.

WORKOUT SIX
CIRCUIT TRAINING

Circuit training is a non-stop programme that alternates between strength and cardiovascular exercises. The cardiovascular work increases the heart rate, helping to pump the blood round the body, before you do some strengthening work. Circuit training is a great way to build strength and endurance, and increase your cardiovascular activity in a short amount of time. You can do a quick 10-minute blast, or a longer 45-minute session by simply repeating the programme two to four times. Whatever your level you can work at your own pace because circuit programmes generally have a time limit for each exercise rather than a fixed number of repetitions. Circuit training requires minimum space and is therefore great for a workout at home.

Because you will only be working on each exercise for a short time you should aim to do them at maximum effort. When you work over long periods of time the body adjusts its breathing patterns to allow you to keep up a steady performance – this is aerobic training. When activity is performed in short, intense bursts a sudden increase of power is required. The body cannot sustain this level of intensity for very long and this type of exercise is called anaerobic.

Hand weights are used for many of these exercises and you can make them at home by using two water-filled bottles or, to make them heavier, fill an empty bottle with sugar to the required weight.

Warm-up: 5 minutes of mobility exercises (see pages 96–7) followed by 5 minutes of cardiovascular exercise, gradually increasing in intensity (see pages 106–111).

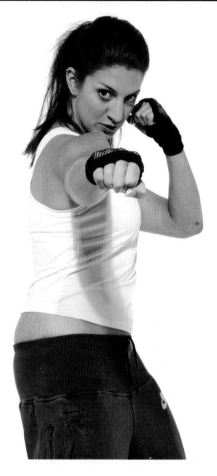

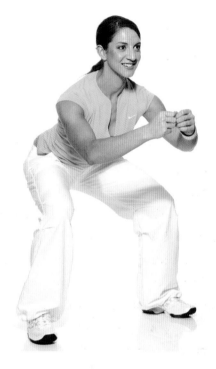

Cardiovascular

To refresh your memory of these exercises see pages 112–121.

- knee lifts – 1 minute
- jab then hook – 1 minute
- scissors – 1 minute
- jab then hook – 1 minute (opposite side)

Time: 4 minutes

Wide Squats

Stand with the feet slightly wider than hips and the knees in line with the second toe. Keep the weight in the heels and think of the chest lifting as you bend the knees, then send the tailbone (the last bone in your spine) backwards while maintaining a flat back. Breathe out as you return to standing, slightly squeezing the abdominals and gluteals as you lift the body.

Sets: 1 x 1 minute
Muscles worked: quads, gluteals, hamstrings

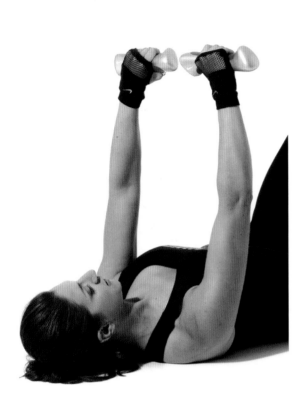

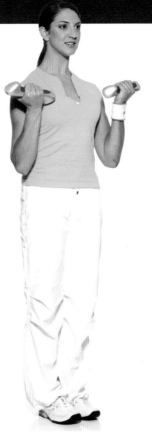

Chest Press

Lie on your back with the knees bent and feet
flat on the floor, parallel with the hips. Hold
a weight in each hand, and have the elbows
on the floor at chest level with the palms
facing forwards, knuckles pointing towards
the ceiling. Keeping the elbows in line with
the wrists, push both hands up and extend the
arms over the centre of the chest, lower them
down and lightly touch the elbows to the floor
before the next repetition.

Sets: 1 x 1 minute
Muscles worked: pectorals, triceps

Biceps Curl

Stand with your feet shoulder-distance apart,
with a weight in each hand and your arms by
your sides. Your hands should face forward.
Keeping the elbows in to the sides, bend them
and lift the weights. Do not swing the trunk
as you lift. Lower the arms back to the sides.
Keep the elbows soft.

Sets: 1 x 1 minute
Muscles worked: biceps

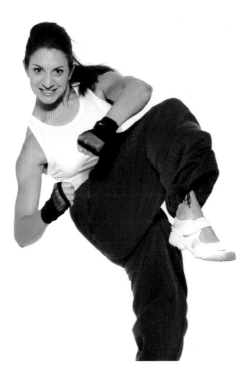

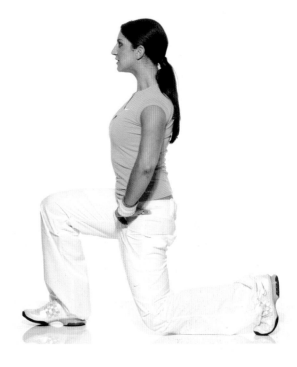

Cardiovascular

- knee lifts – 1 minute
- jab then hook – 1 minute
- scissors – 1 minute
- jab then hook – 1 minute (opposite side)

Time: 4 minutes

Lunges

Stand with feet hip-width apart, with one foot forward and one back. Lift the heel of the back foot. Lower the body down (not forwards) until you adopt a right angle with the back knee (your front knee should bend so your knee is above the ankle – NOT over the toe). Straighten back to the starting position.

Sets: 1 x 1 minute
Muscles worked: quads, hamstrings, gluteals

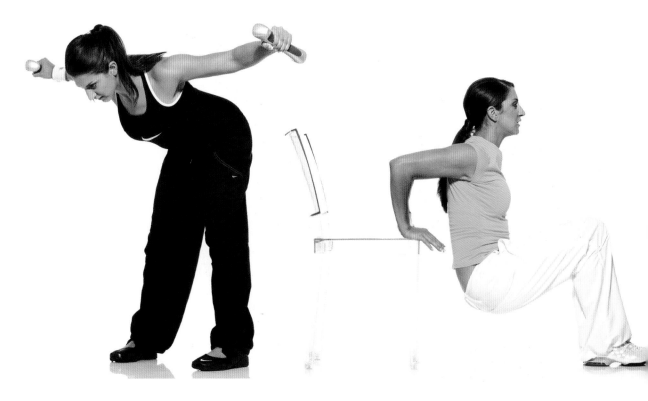

Bent Over Reverse Flies

Have a weight in each hand. Draw the navel to the spine, keep the back straight and lean forward from hips. Arms are lengthened down to the floor and palms facing inwards. Raise the weights out to the side to shoulder height, nip the shoulder blades together, then return the arms to the starting position. You can do this in a seated position if you think you will put too much strain on the back (see page 123).

Sets: 1 x 1 minute
Muscles worked: trapezius

Triceps Dips

Place a chair against a wall and sit on it with your knees bent and feet hip-distance apart. Have your hands on the edge of the chair with the fingers pointing forward. Straighten the arms to lift the bottom up away from the chair. Bend the elbows directly behind you to lower the body, then push through the arms to lift back up. Do not push up using the gluteals – you should feel this in the back of the arms.

Sets: 1 x 1 minute
Muscles worked: triceps

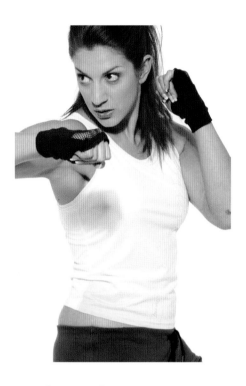

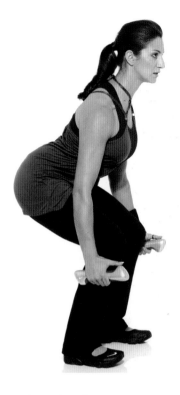

Cardiovascular

- knee lifts – 1 minute
- jab then hook – 1 minute
- scissors – 1 minute
- jab then hook – 1 minute (opposite side)

Time: 4 minutes

Weighted Squats

Stand with the feet slightly wider than the hips and the knees in line with the second toe. Keep the weight in the heels and think of the chest lifting as you bend the knees. Send the tailbone (the last bone in your spine) backwards while maintaining a flat back. Breathe out as you return to standing, slightly squeezing the abdominals and gluteals as you lift the body.

Sets: 1 x 1 minute
Muscle worked: quads, hamstrings and gluteals

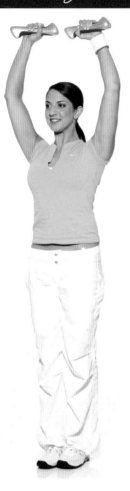

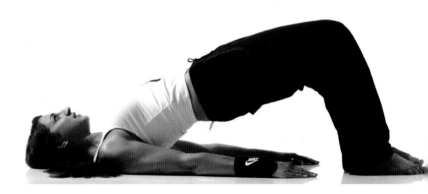

Weighted Shoulder Press

Start with a weight in each hand and arms at shoulder height. Keep the elbows underneath the wrists. Push the weights up above the head and slightly in front (so you can see your hands at all times), don't lock the elbows. Return to the starting position.

Sets: 1 x 1 minute
Muscles worked: shoulders

Hip Lift

Lie on your back with the knees bent, feet flat on the floor, and feet and knees parallel with the hips. The arms are on the floor by the sides. Engage the abdominals and squeeze the bottom as you push towards the ceiling lifting the hips away from the floor. Lower back down with control.

Sets: 1 x 1 minute
Muscles worked: abdominals and gluteals

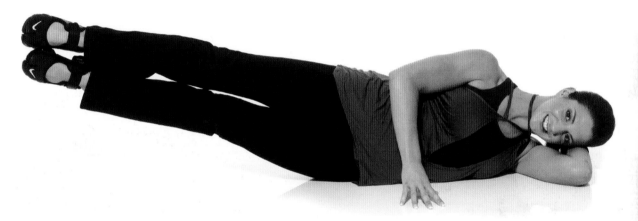

Cardiovascular

- knee lifts – 1 minute
- jab then hook – 1 minute
- scissors – 1 minute
- jab then hook – 1 minute (opposite side)

Time: 4 minutes

Double Leg Lift

Lie on your side, shoulders and hips stacked, keep the legs straight, one on top of the other, feet slightly in front of the hips. Pull in the abdominals, squeeze the legs together and lift them off the floor. Lower with control. A set here is just one lift on one side. Do the repetitions on one side first and then your rest period is the time it takes to turn onto the other side to repeat on that side.

Sets: 1 x 1 minute
Muscles worked: abdominals, abductors, adductors

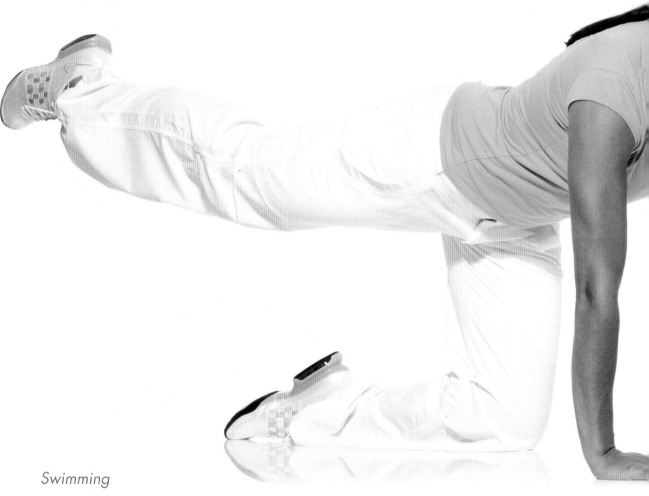

Swimming

Get on all fours in a table-top position (back flat, hands underneath the shoulders and knees underneath the hips). Draw the navel to the spine to prepare. Breathe in, then breathe out as you lengthen and extend opposite arm and leg, maintaining a flat back and without dipping or lifting the shoulders or hips (keep the weight central and don't transfer all the weight onto one side of hip). Breathe in to return smoothly to the starting position. Repeat on the other side.

Sets: 1 x 1 minute
Muscles worked: abdominals, gluteals

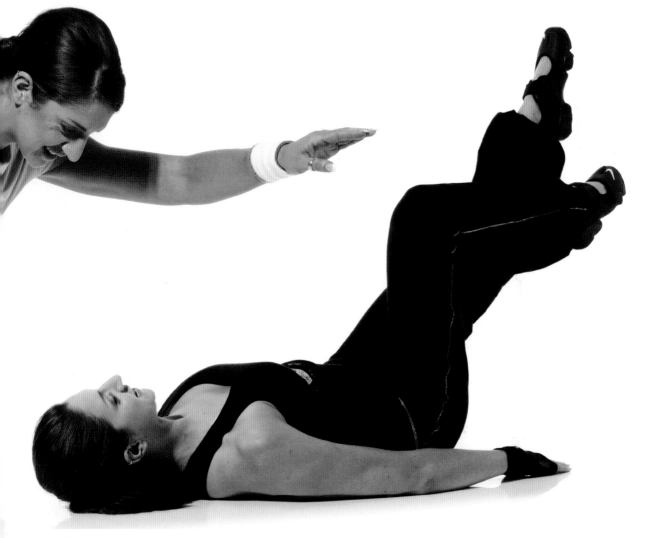

Leg Extensions

Lie on your back with the knees bent at right angles above the hips.
Breathe in to prepare. Breathe out and pull the navel to the spine as
you extend one leg away from you – do NOT allow the back to arch or
abdominals to dome. Breathe in as you bring the knee back to its starting
position. Repeat on the opposite side.

Sets: 1 x 1 minute
Muscles worked: abdominals

Finish with the stretches on page 84–7.

WORKOUT SEVEN
EXPRESS CIRCUIT FOR UPPER BODY
(5–15 Minutes)

Workouts seven, eight and nine are quick workouts you can fit in to your spare moments and do two or three times over, depending on the time you have available. You still need to warm-up first – you can do the first round of exercises at an easy pace as the warm-up – and cool down afterwards. You will still need to do your 30 minutes of activity, including some cardiovascular work at another time in the day.

Hand weights are used for many of these exercises and you can make them at home by using two water-filled bottles or, to make them heavier, fill an empty bottle with sugar to the required weight.

Press-Ups
Start on all fours, with your hands wider than your shoulders, fingers pointing forwards. Engage your abdominals and lower the chest to the floor, bending the elbows as you breathe in. Breathe out, engage the abdominals as you push the hands into the floor to lift the body back up. A full press-up is one with the legs stretched out behind you and toes tucked underneath.

Sets: 1 x 1 minute
Muscles worked: chest, triceps, abdominals

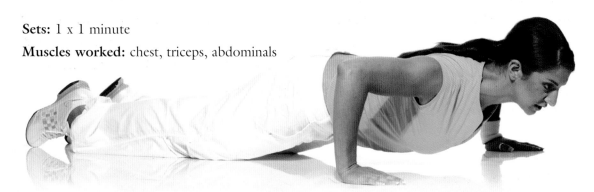

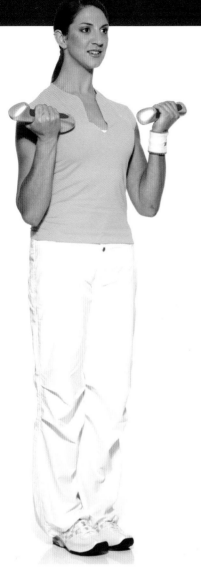

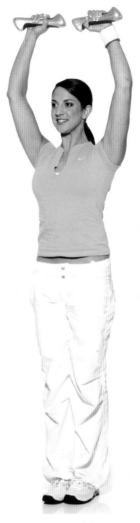

Biceps Curl

Stand with your feet shoulder-distance apart,
with a weight in each hand and your arms by
your sides. Your hands should face forward.
Keeping the elbows in to the sides, bend them
to lift the weights. Do not swing the trunk
as you lift. Lower the arms back to the sides.
Keep the elbows soft.

Sets: 1 x 1 minute
Muscles worked: biceps

Weighted Shoulder Press

Start with a weight in each hand and arms
at shoulder height. Keep the elbows
underneath the wrists. Push up above the head
but slightly in front (so you can see your hands
at all times), don't lock the elbows. Return to
the starting position.

Sets: 1 x 1 minute
Muscles worked: shoulders

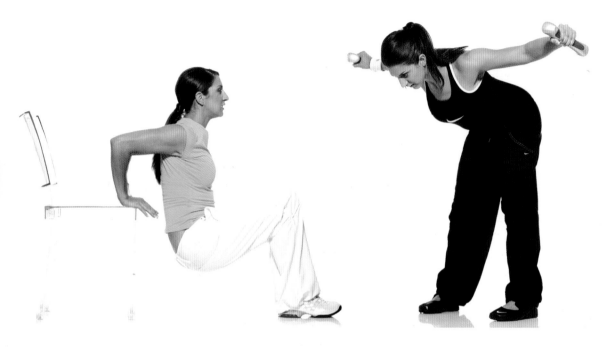

Triceps Dips

Place a chair against a wall and sit on it with your knees bent and feet hip-distance apart. Have your hands on the edge of the chair with the fingers pointing forward. Straighten the arms to lift the bottom up away from the chair. Bend the elbows directly behind you to lower the body, then push through the arms to lift back up. Do not push up using the gluteals – you should feel this in the back of the arms.

Sets: 1 x 1 minute
Muscles worked: triceps

Bent Over Reverse Flies

Have a weight in each hand. Draw the navel to the spine, keep the back straight and lean forward from hips. Arms are lengthened down to the floor and palms facing inwards. Raise the weights out to the side to shoulder height, nip the shoulder blades together, then return the arms to the starting position. You can do this in a seated position if you think you will put too much strain on the back (see page 123).

Sets: 1 x 1 minute
Muscles worked: upper back/shoulders

Here is a series of stretches to finish off with which are designed specifically to stretch the muscles you have been working. Hold the stretches for 10 to 15 seconds.

Upper Back Stretch

Clasp the hands in front of the body. Round the back, don't lock out the elbows, and gently pull the arms forward and drop the chin to the chest.

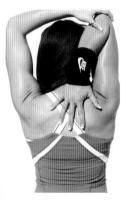

Triceps Stretch

Lift one arm and place the other hand on the elbow. Bend the arm so the hand is coming down between the shoulder blades. Gently push the arm back with the other hand until you feel a stretch in the back of the upper arm.

Or, you can take one arm across the body, put one hand just below the elbow and ease the arm further across. Release and change arms.

Biceps Stretch

Open the arms to the sides and point the thumbs down. Continue to push the thumbs down as you reach the arms back until you feel a stretch on the front of the upper arm.

Or, you can take one arm in front of you with the palm facing upwards. Press downwards with the other hand into the palm of the raised hand, release and change arms.

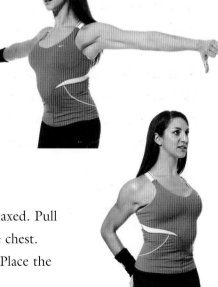

Chest Stretch

Place both hands in the small of the back. Keep the shoulders relaxed. Pull the elbows backwards until you feel a sufficient stretch across the chest.

Or, turn and face a wall and lift one arm to shoulder height. Place the hand on the wall and slowly turn the body away from the arm.

WORKOUT EIGHT
EXPRESS CIRCUIT FOR LEGS AND BOTTOM
(5–15 Minutes)

Warm-up: see workout seven on page 178.

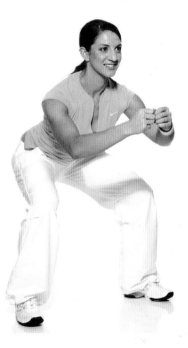

Wide Squats

Stand with the feet slightly wider than the hips and the knees in line with the second toe. Keep the weight in the heels and think of the chest lifting as you bend the knees, then send the tailbone (the last bone in your spine) backwards while maintaining a flat back. Breathe out as you return to standing, slightly squeezing the abdominals and gluteals as you lift the body.

Sets: 1 x 1 minute
Muscles worked: quads, gluteals, hamstrings

Inner Thigh Lift

Lie on your side with the top leg bent slightly forwards, resting the knee on the floor in front of you. Keep the toes pointing forwards as you lift and lower the underneath leg.

Sets: 1 x 1 minute
Muscles worked: adductors

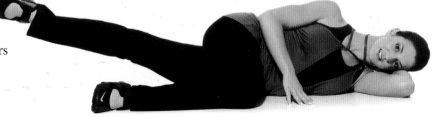

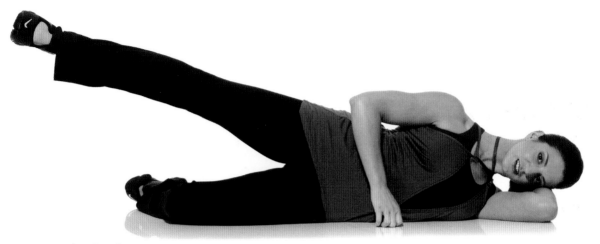

Outer Thigh Lift

Lie on your side with the underneath leg bent slightly forward and the top leg extended. Keep the toes pointing forward as you lift and lower the upper leg.

Sets: 1 x 1 minute
Muscles worked: abductors

Hip Lift

Lie on your back with the knees bent, feet flat on the floor, and feet and knees parallel with the hips. The arms are on the floor by the sides. Engage the abdominals and squeeze the bottom as you push towards the ceiling lifting the hips away from the floor. Lower back down with control.

Sets: 1 x 1 minute
Muscles worked: abdominals and gluteals

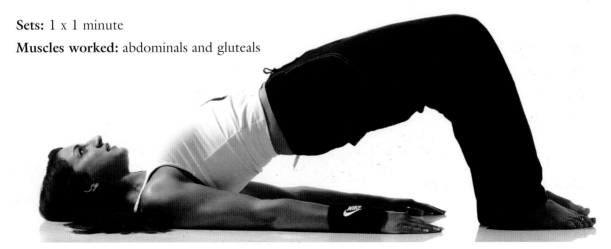

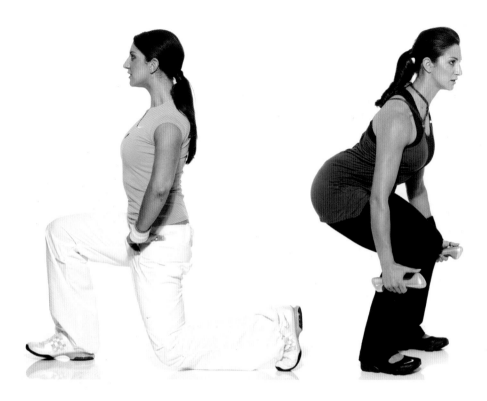

Lunges

Stand with the feet hip-width apart, with one foot in front of the other. Lift the heel of the back foot. Lower the body down (not forwards) until you are at a right angle with the back knee (your front knee should bend so your knee is above the ankle – NOT over the toe). Return to the starting position. Repeat starting with the other leg in front.

Sets: 1 x 1 minute
Muscles worked: quads, gluteals, hamstrings

Weighted Squats

Hold a weight in each hand and stand with the feet slightly wider than the hips. The feet should be parallel and the toes pointing forward. Keep the weight in the heels and think of the chest lifting as you bend the knees. Send the tailbone (the last bone in your spine) backwards while maintaining a flat back. Breathe out as you return to standing, slightly squeezing the abdominals and gluteals as you lift the body.

Sets: 1 x 1 minute
Muscles worked: quads, gluteals, hamstrings

Here is a series of stretches to finish off with which are designed specifically to stretch the muscles you have been working. Hold the stretches for between 30 and 45 seconds.

Quad Stretch

Stand on one foot and hold the other foot in your hand – hold on to something if you need to. Keep the knees soft. Draw the knee up and the foot back towards the spine until you feel a stretch in the front of the thigh. You can do this stretch lying on one side with your knees bent up in line with the hips. Hold the ankle of the top leg and, keeping the leg bent, draw it back so the knee is moving towards the spine. Stop when you get a stretch. Repeat on the other side.

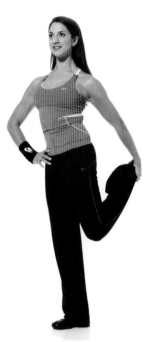

Hamstring Stretch

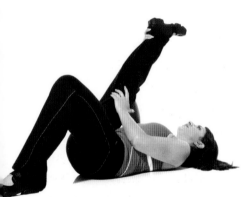

Lie on your back with knees bent, feet flat on the floor. Lift one leg and put one hand behind the knee (do NOT hold onto the kneecap) and the other hand behind your ankle. Straighten the leg until you feel a stretch at the back of the thigh. Try and ease the stretch a little further, release, and change legs.

Calf Stretch

Stand with both hips and feet facing forwards. Step back with one foot, shift your weight forward so the front leg bends slightly and the upper body comes in line with the back leg. Keep the back heel down on the floor. You should feel the stretch in the back leg. Release and change legs.

WORKOUT NINE
EXPRESS CIRCUIT FOR ABDOMINALS
(5–15 Minutes)

Warm-up: see workout seven on page 178.

Abdominal Crunch

Lie flat on your back with your legs and feet slightly wider than your hips. Place your hands behind the head to support it. On no account pull on the head. Breathe out and draw the abdominals in, navel to spine, and curl the upper body up off the floor. Aim to draw the ribcage down towards the hips so that the abdominal wall contracts flat and compact – don't let the abdominals dome. Keep a small gap between the chin and the chest. Breathe in to lower yourself back to the starting position.

Sets: 1 x 1 minute
Muscles worked: abdominals

Oblique Twist and Reach

Lie flat on your back with your legs and feet slightly wider than your hips. Place one hand behind the head to support it. Do not pull on the head. Breathe out and draw the abdominals in, navel to spine, and lift the upper body. Aim to draw the ribcage down towards the hips so that the abdominal wall contracts flat and compact – don't let the abdominals dome and keep a small gap between the chin and the chest. Reach the free arm over to the opposite knee, aiming to take the shoulder away from the floor as you twist across the body. Breathe in to lower.

Sets: 1 x 1 minute
Muscles worked: abdominals-obliques

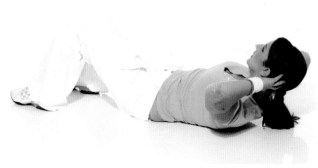

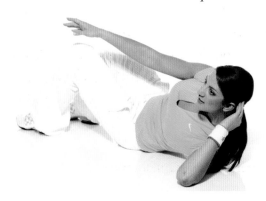

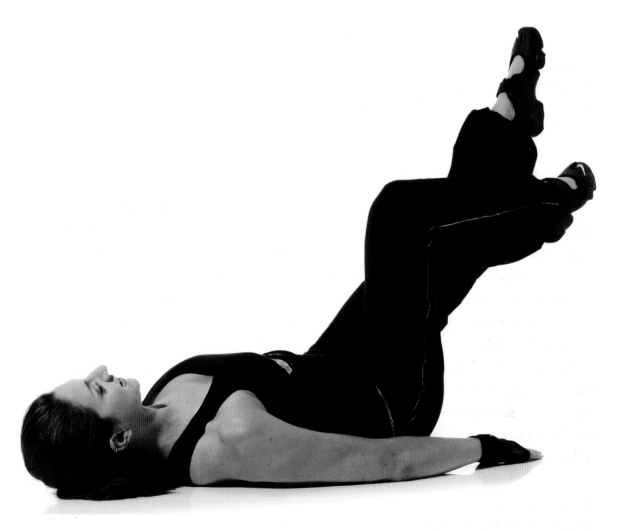

Leg Extensions

Lie on your back with the knees bent at a right angle above the
hips. Breathe in to prepare. Breathe out, draw navel to spine as you
extend one leg away from you – do NOT allow the back to arch or
the abdominals to dome. Breathe in as you return the foot back to
its starting position, then repeat on opposite side.

Sets: 1 x 1 minute
Muscles worked: abdominals

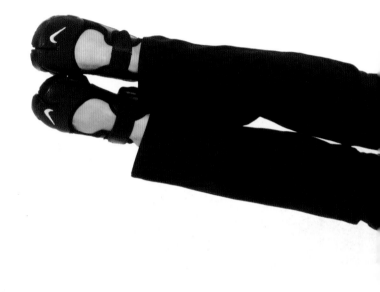

Reverse Sit Up (Roll Down)

Sit upright on your sitting bones (right at the bottom of your pelvis). You can have your knees bent or legs straight in front of you. Keep the legs together. Pull in your abdominals and tuck the pelvis underneath you as you slowly roll down towards the floor to a position where you feel your abdominals contract effectively without any doming. Keep your back curved as you go down and come up.

Sets: 1 x 1 minute
Muscle worked: abdominals

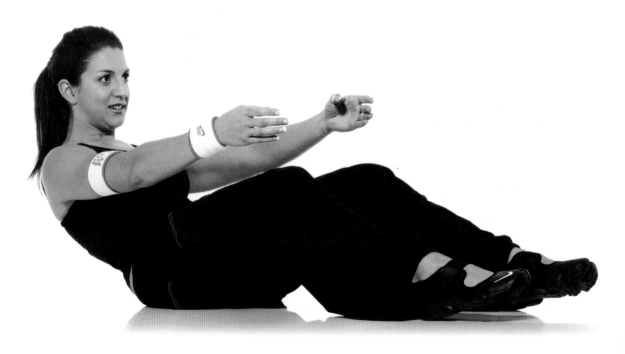

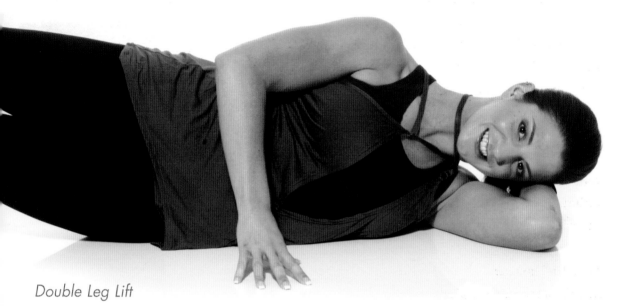

Double Leg Lift

Lie on your side, shoulders and hips stacked, keep th legs straight, one n top of the other, feet slightly in front of the hips. Pull in the abdominals and lift both legs together. Lower with control. Repeat on the other side.

Sets: 1 x 1 minute
Muscles worked: abdominals, adductors, abductors

To finish off this workout, lie on your back and stretch your arms and legs away from your centre to release the abdominals, then release. Repeat this a couple of times.

You could also roll onto your front, position the hands on the floor slightly above the head and push down through the forearms to lift the torso, again releasing the abdominals but taking care not to over extend the back too much.

COOL DOWN

After stretching to cool down, a relaxation is a very good way of finishing off your workout, or indeed if you feel particularly stressed after a bad day!

How Do I Achieve Relaxed Muscles?

Progressive muscular relaxation involves actively contracting and relaxing them. When a muscle is tightened for 4 to 6 seconds and then released, it returns to a more relaxed state. This should be performed for the following parts of the body in turn – feet, legs, thighs, buttocks, stomach, back, neck, shoulders, arms, hands, jaw, face and eyes.

Relaxation Position

You may choose to get into this position before you exercise in order to prepare the mind for the exercise you are about to take, or last thing in the evening to help you sleep better, or at any point through the day when you feel the need to unwind and gather your thoughts. It will help you relax any tense muscles as well as lengthening the spine and widening and relaxing the torso.

- Lie on your back with your knees bent, feet flat on the floor, hip- or shoulder-distance apart. Keep your knees in line with your toes.
- Make sure your neck is tension free. Your nose should be level with your chin (you may need someone to check this for you at first). In some cases the chin can be higher and in this situation you should place a small pillow under the head for the neck to be fully lengthened and comfortable.
- Place your hands on the lower abdominal area so they form a triangle pointing towards the pubic bone. The heels of the hand should be perched on the hip bones and the fingers on the pubic bone. Rock the pelvis so you can feel how your fingers lift higher than your thumbs

and your thumbs higher than your fingers as you tilt your pelvis gently forward and backward. Find a position where your hands are lying flat.

- Keep your hands on the abdomen for the initial awareness of your breathing.
- Breathe in and feel your torso lengthen and your ribcage lift.
- Breathe out and allow your shoulders to soften, drop and open.
- Breathe in wide.
- Breathe out and let your shoulders relax some more.
- Breathe in and focus on your ribcage.
- Breathe out and feel your ribcage soften and relax down towards the floor. As you breathe think of the ribcage melting down into the floor.
- Breathe in.
- Breathe out and focus on releasing inner tension.
- Breathe in.
- Breathe out and feel the hips softening.

You can spend as long as you need in this position, focusing on any specific area of your body that is particularly tense. Use each exhalation to release and let go, feel your body getting rid of any tension and melting into the floor. This is a great thinking position and a place to gather your thoughts in times of stress. Remember that stress generally builds upwards through the back, which is why we notice it more in the shoulders. It's time to let go in this simple exercise.

5
POSITIVE
POSTURE

many of us are considered to have poor posture. In fact, every one of us has developed strong posture for the needs of the jobs we undertake every day. Your body has developed or adapted over time to sitting at a desk, or standing poorly and the unfortunate result of moving from the 'correct alignment' our bodies were designed with is that we notice pain, injuries and change of shape. For example, people who spend a lot of time at a computer or desk may find they have round shoulders. Around 70 per cent of people at work suffer discomfort or pain, usually in the back. Sitting incorrectly or for too long without a break increases the chance of developing repetitive strain injury (RSI) and other soft tissue injuries. The more you choose to ignore these problems or don't take enough breaks to stretch or change position the more difficult they become to correct.

Ideal posture should allow all joints to be in a neutral position (not forced too much in one direction or restricted in any way, which may cause an imbalance). Imagine a plumb line going through the centre of your body from top to toe. It should go down the body from the top of your head and pass:

- at a right angle with the earlobes
- parallel with the centre of the neck
- at a right angle with the tips of the shoulders
- through the ribcage, dividing it in half
- parallel with the lumbar vertebrae
- slightly behind the hip joint
- slightly in front of the knee joint
- slightly in front of the outer edge of the ankle bone

External factors such as hereditary genetic disorders, illness and even the sports you play may also cause a change in your posture. The environment in which you work or live will have an impact. These factors can lead to injury or imbalances that will increase as your body adapts to your lifestyle. Concentration and awareness are needed to correct poor posture.

There are three main incorrect posture types:

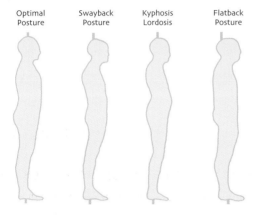

| Optimal | Swayback | Kyphosis | Flatback |
| Posture | Posture | Lordosis | Posture |

THE SWAYBACK

This slouching posture is commonly seen in teenagers! The head is forward, the upper back appears long and the spine is swayed backwards. The pelvis sways forward in relation to the feet. Your hamstrings at the back of the thigh and some of your abdominals will be strong, while your back and neck muscles will be weak.

KYPHOSIS LORDOSIS

The head is thrust forward, there is curvature to the upper back and an arching of the lower back causing the pelvis to tilt forward. The abdominals are prone to weakness and the knees may hyperextend.

THE FLATBACK

The head is again forward, the upper back is rounded slightly but the lower section is quite straight. The hamstrings and abdominals may be strong and the muscles in the front of the hips weak.

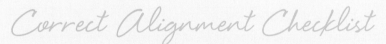

Correct Alignment Checklist

- Allow your head to go forward and up slightly.
- The neck should be relaxed. Your ears should be aligned with the tops of your shoulders.
- Keep your shoulder blades down and back. Don't confuse this with sticking your chest out. Imagine a triangle shape in your upper back and feel as though you are drawing your shoulder blades down towards your waist and back in a 'V'.
- Keep your breastbone soft – imagine having two small buckles attaching the bottom of the ribcage to your hips.
- Lengthen up through the spine – imagine you are being pulled up by a cord running through your centre. It's giving you instant height and reducing the compression of each vertebrae. The cord keeps you feeling tall while also allowing your body to be tension free.
- Check your pelvis is in a neutral position – not tilting forward or backward, but still keeping a small curve in your lower back. Try rocking the pelvis forward and backward, so your lower spine flattens and curves; this should help you understand your body's natural movement. Repeat this movement a few times and once you are comfortable settle in to a place that is in-between, neither too arched nor too flat.
- Knees are soft but not bent – you need to have relaxed knees to allow movement in your pelvis.
- Feet should be hip or shoulder distance apart and parallel, keep the weight evenly on each foot and don't roll them in or out.

GETTING YOUR POSTURE RIGHT

To determine your posture type, get someone to take a picture of you or use a tripod. Stand barefoot near a straight wall in a relaxed position that is natural to you. Wear a swimsuit or tight clothing to reveal the outline of your body. Date the picture for reference. You can take more pictures at regular intervals to the changes in your posture as you progress.

To find a good standing position, sway very gently forward and backward keeping the body in one straight line. What do you feel? You want to have the weight of the body equally on three points of the foot – big toe, little toe and heel. Try to find this position while keeping the body straight.

Hopefully your awareness should also be drawn to your abdominal area. Notice how your stomach muscles are more noticeably activated when you are at the extreme end of the sway forward and backward. This is your body naturally increasing the contraction of the muscles as a response (as if in preparation for a fall) to your movement. Bring your weight back to the centre until you feel equally balanced on all three points of the foot again and be aware of your abdominal tension, keeping engaged at a level where you can breathe easily.

Read through the correct alignment checklist again and perform the exercise in front of the mirror and you will see an immediate improvement. Hold the position for at least 5 minutes, then relax and read on.

Firstly, how did you feel standing with correct posture? Hopefully, seeing the effect in the mirror should have made you feel good. But what about after you had held the new position for a while? How did you feel then? Slightly uneasy and uncomfortable? Finally, what happened when you relaxed? Did you all of a sudden let everything go and return to a slouched or poorer postural position?

If holding the position was pretty easy and you didn't make too many changes when you relaxed then great, but if you noticed a lot of change and deterioration in your posture with release or it was uncomfortable to hold the correct position for too long, it is time to start realizing that you are spending the majority of your time in a bad position and clearly getting better at it!

So how are you going to take your first steps to change? It's not going to happen overnight. You have spent the majority of your life growing into the position you are currently in. With a steady approach and constant improvements and amendments your posture will become the best it possibly can be. The result: not only will you look good – you will feel great.

Let's look at ways in which to tweak your posture with subtle changes which are easy to remember and will have a huge impact on the way that you look and feel. Practising this on a regular basis will form a new habit that strengthens and continually improves. You will have to constantly remind yourself what to do in the beginning but over time it will become an unconscious adjustment.

Remember the exercise we did on page 4 to lose a few centimetres immediately? All we did was to lengthen, grow and draw the navel towards the spine into a position which allowed us to breathe normally. Here's another example. When you are planning an important evening out in your favourite outfit, step out of the shower, put your underwear on and stand in front of the mirror … now, how do you stand? All squashed down, without a care, portraying a bad image? Or do you pull up and in and try to look your best? But when you have put on your outfit and you give yourself that final once-over before you go downstairs to greet whoever may be waiting, do you pull up, pull in, maybe twirl to view your other angles then walk with elegance, confidence and grace? If you look good, chances are you may get a compliment. Was it your favourite outfit that made you feel like this, or was it, in fact, you? With your confidence you have carried yourself with poise, looked important and the positive image you are portraying is obvious to others.

So how are you going to make this position become your normal one? Put yourself in an everyday situation that may take 10 minutes or so, watering the garden, for example, or going to the supermarket. Now, what I want you to do is perform that daily routine and pull your abdominals in by 30 per cent before you start the activity. I often suggest to my clients they imagine being in their underwear – 'naked shopping' I call it – and in an instant people pull up and in – they know exactly what I mean! Try this and see how quickly you get used to it. At first you will have to concentrate but it will become automatic as your body gently adapts. Before you know it you will be walking or maybe 'strutting' like it's Friday night every night.

The 30% Rule: pull your abs in by 30% when you carry out daily tasks: it will make all the difference!

I often used to sit with my boyfriend in coffee shops and 'people watch' – if you have never done this, you should. It is so interesting to watch busy people and see a few seconds of their life as they walk past you. One particular morning we were sitting quietly and he said, 'Great walk.' My first thought was, 'Must be a gorgeous girl with legs up to her armpits … OK, I'll look.' And I looked up and my eyes were drawn to the same person in an instant. Not the stereotype I had conjured up in my head, just a normal woman who looked amazing, so confident that she stood out from the crowd. A great walk she certainly had and her positive body image almost created a glow around her. It does not take much to recognize your bad posture habits and slowly begin to correct them – and you'll get the same result as that woman.

FINDING THE POSITION OF A LIFETIME

Imagine wearing a huge weightlifter's belt so thick you immediately have to lift your ribcage from your hips (instant height fix). The belt has ten notches on it.

- By drawing the navel into the spine (imagine you have a piece of string attached to your navel which is pulling your stomach towards your back) pull your stomach in by 100 per cent or to belt notch ten – then release.
- Now try the same thing, but draw in to around belt notch seven or eight (70 to 80 per cent).
- Now just draw in to notch five (50 per cent).
- Now come to just below that position at belt notch three (30 per cent).

This is the position you should try to hold while you move about in every-day life. There should be no unnecessary tension in the shoulders and you should be able to breathe comfortably. You should just be aware of using your abdominals. You are almost mimicking how you would feel if you were wearing a basque or a corset as they did in Victorian times. The muscles are slightly activated providing you with extra support as you move. Did you ever see a Victorian lady walk with bad posture? Maintaining this position will make you less prone to injury; you may be aware of the muscles getting a little tighter during some movements, acting as a layer of protection. Try and increase the intensity of this contraction when you might need it more, for example when you are about to lift the shopping bags, pull your stomach in by 50 or 60 per cent.

Celebrities generally look great when pictured in magazines. They learn to work with their bodies and pose for the camera standing still or taking the walk on the red carpet. Now you can too!

PICTURE PERFECT

Ever wondered why it is that some people always look great in photographs and others don't? It's nothing to do with the camera, it's to do with the way you act in front of it.

Take a closer look at how the celebrities stand, hold themselves and even what expression they pull … any seem familiar?

Cheryl Tweedy often has a glowing, wide smile and stands with her weight slightly on the back foot and her right hand on her hip. Victoria Beckham often has a sexy pout and a lengthened pose with legs together and one knee slightly soft, pointing in towards the body. Coleen shows off her great smile and also often stands with one hand on her hip with the weight

Tips for Top Posture

- Do be aware of how you sit – don't slouch, use your core to sit straight.
- Do carry weights such as shopping bags evenly on both sides of the body.
- When carrying children use your core muscles and don't have the baby always on the same hip.
- Swap the receiver of the phone over regularly to avoid neck tension.
- Change your shoes often – they can determine how you walk. Avoid constantly wearing high heels.
- Sit at a PC square on.
- When bending down, bend your knees and keep your tummy tucked in.
- Go 'naked shopping' or do other activities with the abdominals engaged.
- Observe your body posture in front of the mirror regularly – correct it and try and maintain the good position.
- Stretch whenever you feel a tension build-up if you have been sitting for a while.

slightly on the back foot. Paris Hilton is known for a subtle pursed-kiss pout while slightly looking over her shoulder.

I'm sure you would agree, there is rarely a bad picture of any of these celebrities and if there is it is only because they have been caught off guard. Now it's time to bring out the celebrity in you. As you learn how to hold a better posture you should be able to notice the difference in your appearance in the mirror. Each time you get dressed I want you to treat your clothes as your 'best outfit', even if it is your jogging bottoms!

How To Do It!

Look in the mirror, really look, and hold the pose where you look your best. Set up a tripod, if you have one, or get a camera you can put somewhere to get a few body shots. Remember, what you see in the mirror is only a reflection, so it's time to get happy with that picture-perfect pose. Don't treat this as a 'vain campaign' this is simply an exercise you will have to do only once in order to get the picture you will start using for ever! When you have taken a few shots look through them – don't mock them and be negative, turn the worst one upside down, then use your positive voice to extract the flattering parts from each shot. Now, take a few more shots trying to recapture only the best bits; take another look and repeat as many times as you need until you feel you have a good average shot. Do the same with a head shot, try different angles allowing you to see each side of your face to establish your best side! The more you practise and become familiar and comfortable with the camera the more your natural confidence will flow and you will really begin to own the picture. Select your best picture so far, turn over the worst picture and hold them side by side. See the difference.

You have not had to lose weight, get changed or put extra make-up on to look like this, you have simply learnt to use your body to its best advantage. Now go out there and look like your best picture.

6
REWARDS AND FEEL-GOOD FIXES

REWARDS

It is important that you reward yourself for your achievements regularly. Think of all the things you like doing or you consider a treat. Write a list and categorize them into big or little. The big rewards should be taken when you have reached a target you have set yourself and might be anything from buying a new outfit to a spa treatment – just make sure it is something you would really look forward to having as a prize reward. The smaller ones will be weekly rewards for your commitment and efforts.

If your big target is weight loss, don't weigh yourself every day. Do it weekly in the morning and record your weight. As you begin to tone up your body you may find you do not actually lose weight according to the scales because your fat is changing into muscle and muscle is heavier than fat. Take your body measurements for an accurate record of your changes and see how your clothes fit. Your first big goal might be to get into a particular outfit, for example. It's important to remember that the main goals are not going to be reached overnight and with this in mind the smaller rewards are essential for making you feel positive and focused on reaching the next level.

Think about the small rewards, the things you can look forward to or the things that are purely based on 'you time'. It can be anything from reading a book, getting a haircut or time-out 'icing on the cake' home beauty treatments – things that will allow you to feel good but, more importantly, are for you and no one else. First I want you to almost strip yourself of the small luxuries you might normally have or take for granted. Put them back in place as a small reward and make yourself work for them.

Reward yourself with fabulous treats – after all your hard work you deserve it!

Tips to Keep On Track

- Wake up with energy. Think about what you are going to achieve during the day before you even move. Think about what makes you happy, then smile! Set the alarm a little earlier if need be. An alarm bell should be a wonderful sound announcing a new day and new adventures! Wake up to music on the radio to get you dancing or chat to make you laugh.
- Sing in the shower and moisturize well using your favourite oils or lotions and put some perfume on.
- Eat a good breakfast – and enjoy it.
- At times when you feel the need for chocolate, cigarettes or anything you are trying to stay away from, go for a brisk walk or a run. A breath of fresh air and some pulse raising activity will make you feel a whole lot better – and could be put towards a mini reward for your success in not giving in!
- Stay positive. Negative attitudes will make it harder to reach your goals. If you believe you will succeed, you will.
- Get enough sleep. Fatigue can have a negative effect on your attitude, and you need to feel good for your positive wake up!

MAGICAL FEEL-GOOD FIXES

Why do we feel so good after exercise? Tests have shown that the chemical beta endorphin, released by the pituitary gland during activity, gives the body a feeling of happiness, even euphoria and eliminates pain and stress while also delaying the signs of ageing! So exercising on its own is a really feel-good fix. Here are a few beauty ideas to give you a different sort of feel-good fix.

Moisturizing all parts of your body is a must and makes your skin feel smooth and supple. Moisturize your face every day, using a cream with a decent UV and sun protection factor and don't forget your lips – they may chap in outdoor weather conditions. Step up your moisturizing if you are showering more or training outdoors. And don't forget your feet, they need moisturizing regularly – and exfoliate them every couple of weeks to prevent any build up of hard skin.

Here are some oils you can mix yourself to give you a quick feel-good fix. Using a base of organic grapeseed or sweet almond oil, add the following:

- To hydrate: 1 drop ylang ylang, 2 drops bergamot, 3 drops sandalwood.
- To relieve tired/aching muscles: put 3 drops eucalyptus, 2 drops lavender, 1 tablespoon base oil in the water while the bath is running.
- To rejuvenate the face: 1 drop rosewood, 1 drop frankincense in a base oil.
- To relax in your bath: 1 tablespoon base oil, 2 drops lavender, 2 drops chamomile.
- To relieve sinus problems or a cold: 1 tablespoon base oil, 1 teaspoon aloe vera, 1 teaspoon wheatgerm, 2 drops peppermint, 2 drops eucalyptus – rub on to the chest, upper back and neck. Your body will heat the oil and the aroma will clear your sinuses.

A home manicure will also make you feel good and can be done while sitting comfortably on the sofa with a healthy glass of fresh juice! You could use it as a small reward or, if you want a real lift, visiting a salon for a professional treatment could be one of your big rewards.

You'll need some warm olive oil, a nail file, scissors or clippers, cuticle pusher, sanding block (optional), polish (optional).

- Soak your nails in warm olive oil to strengthen them if they are weak or brittle.

- Wash your hands thoroughly and dry them well.
- Trim your nails to the desired length.
- File them to your preferred shape – round, pointed or square.
- Push your cuticles back if you need to and sand any ridges if necessary.
- Apply a clear polish then a colour of your choice.
- If you are doing your toes as well, match fingers and toes with the same colour or opt for a slightly darker shade on your toes.

Eyebrow shaping can make a huge impact on the shape of your face and the appearance of your eyes. Depending upon your skill and confidence you can do it at home or visit a salon. Some home kits come equipped with all the things you need.

- Brush your eyebrows with a comb or a clean mascara brush.
- Line up a stencil of an eyebrow (if in the kit) or draw the desired shape with an eye pencil and tweeze round the shape.
- Buy a natural lash gel to define the shape of your eyelashes.
- Use eyebrow pencil on the brow for final definition if required.

How about a bit of fake tan to make you feel as though you've been on the beach (but without the sunburn!)? A tan makes you look slimmer and healthier – the holiday or sun-kissed look that people often compliment! Fake tans can be a little bit trial and error. You should seek further assistance for a recommended brand that suits your skin tone and offers a good finish. There are creams, mousses and sprays on the market which all promise a streak-free tan. Some develop within hours, while some will require polishing or washing off after a certain time – read the label first! Moisturize all over first and put a little extra on the elbows, knees, ankles and on the undersides of the arms. Apply the fake tan as directed. Lastly, apply a little more moisturizer on the areas mentioned above for optimum no-streak blending. As an alternative and reversible method for a fake tan you can add some foundation to your moisturizer. This will also help hide any marks or blemishes you may have.

Try a new hairstyle. Now, unless a complete hair makeover is one of your big rewards, you can achieve a new look through a simple transformation of your normal style – pinned up, straightened, curled, ringlets, plaits, tied up, bun, chignon … There are many things on the market such as bendy curlers, chignon bases and even false hair that can be clipped in to help transform a plain look into a sophisticated one without too much hassle. Scarves, headbands and clips can also give a subtle well-groomed appearance without breaking the bank. If you are short of ideas or really don't know where to begin, ask your hairdresser for advice or buy a magazine that has easy to follow directions.

It's important to make sure you have a radiant face and a good complexion. As a small reward buy a good brand of cleanser, toner and moisturizer for your face. Exfoliating every other day will clear dead skin cells and you should invest in a facemask or peel as a midweek lift.

These facial exercises will tighten and tone any sagging skin and make you feel really great and glamorous-looking!

- To lift the eyebrows, push the centre of the brows upwards until the skin is taut, then try and close the eyes, hold them shut for 5 seconds and repeat 5–10 times.
- For puffiness underneath the eyes, pull the skin down from the top of the cheekbones and try and close the eyes, hold them shut for 5 seconds and repeat 5–10 times.
- Scrunch the face up then open it wide, purse the lips together then move the jaw to the right, and then the left, smile as widely as you can and release, smile again and tuck the chin in!

- Laugh as much as possible – the more we frown, the more we are improving the frown line ... don't overdo the frowning, increase the smiles. A smile is contagious. Smile at someone and it's more than likely they will smile back. Don't be afraid to pass on a smile!

Feel-Good Fashion

All the small rewards must be designed to give you a positive inner feeling. These are also the small things that may 'top off' the desired look of your bigger goal such as an occasion out where you want to show off the new you in a new outfit. It's a time for you to look and feel amazing ... but don't go wrong by choosing an outfit that doesn't suit you despite you liking it in a magazine. Make the most of your assets by working with your body shape, features and skin tone. Choose colour schemes that complement you. If you are making clothes buying part of your big reward scheme make sure you limit your purchases with a view to achieving further goals and remember that your body shape may continue changing.

Underwear makes a big difference to your final appearance; it can make you appear slimmer and curvier in all the right places. Too many women wear a bra that is the wrong size and does nothing for them. Go to a shop that will measure you properly and remember that your shape changes over time, so have a fitting once every so often. If worn too tight pants cut into the body causing bumps, and wearing the wrong colours can also give the disastrous VPL (visible pantie line). It's much better to opt for a size that is slightly too big for a more flattering fit. We may have laughed at the Bridget Jones style belly warmers, but with the right outfit a fitted corset or brief set can work wonders for a smooth contoured fit. Feel super sexy with matching underwear. Even if it is not seen by a partner it will make you feel more desirable!

Tips to Make the Most of Your Assets

- When buying an item of clothing be sure you have accessories to go with it. Make sure it is multipurpose and will go with several things you already have in your wardrobe to create different looks.
- Petite women should wear fitting clothes or soft flowing lines with narrow belts so as not to shorten their appearance further. Avoid heavy or bold prints. Stripes will elongate the legs.
- Tall women should avoid tight-fitting garments and items that are too long. You can visually reduce your height by wearing tops that are lower than the waistline or wide chunky belts.
- Wide hips should be complemented by lighter shades on top and darker below. Wear V necks, fitted jackets or tops to draw in your waist and give a smooth hour-glass shape. Avoid big loose tops, as this will make you appear wider. Keep skirts knee length.
- If you are large busted, wear long jackets but avoid anything too bold or floaty on top. Darker colours would be a better option and would work well balanced with pleats to bring the eye focus down. V necks are slimming while high or round necks can simply make you look larger. Make sure you wear good underwear.
- If you have a round tummy, wear an empire line to flatter.
- Business clothes can make you look and feel very important. A great suit will last a long time, so make sure you get it right and seek the advice of an assistant or friend to achieve the look that works best for you.

STAY ON TRACK ON HOLIDAY

Here are a few holiday helpers so that you don't backslide during those happy days on the beach or those frantic nights in the night club! Up your workouts for a few weeks before you leave so you really feel your best. Book into a salon or have a bikini and leg wax at home, but make sure you do this a few days before you leave so the skin has chance to calm. And about a week or so before you go start using a fake tan to build a fabulous glow. Ditch the mascara – it's hopeless in the sun – try dying your lashes for a beautiful fresh look.

Make sure you drink plenty of water on the flight and don't drink too much alcohol. Take moisturizer and lip balm on the plane, as it is very easy for the skin to dehydrate.

Pack a selection of ideal holiday exercises like the Pilates programme on page 98 so you can maintain a good posture in your evening outfits, and when you're away make sure you swim or walk and sightsee so you get plenty of daily exercise. Respect your bikini body. Take a high-protection sun block, especially for the face and avoid eating too much wheat, which could make you bloat and feel sluggish.

STAY ON TRACK EVERY DAY

Start the day with a positive thought or saying; write it down and put it somewhere you will see it during the day to improve your smile count! Here are a few examples to get you started:

- You can't have too much of a good thing – so enjoy it.
- Winners do what losers don't want to.

> 'The greatest mistake you can make in life is to be continually fearing you will make one'
>
> *E. Hubbard*
> *1856–1915*

- There are happy feelings and unhappy feelings – choose happy.
- Getting things wrong is simply an elimination process, allowing you to find the best way to do something right.

Smile and the world smiles with you! Being happy makes you smile and feel wonderful. It also allows the world to see you at your best and allows others to catch that contagious happy bug and those energy vibes that you give out. Being optimistic allows you a brighter future and its great advantage is that it can banish or sooth any negative feeling. Studies show that being happy protects you from stress and helps you live longer. Stay focused on being happy by avoiding conflict and sharing understanding. Get on with others and try, when appropriate, to give and receive smiles. By creating a happy environment and making small changes to how you deal with situations in your workplace, home or in the street can make a huge difference to the way people respond to you and feel about themselves.

Happiness is contagious – so go ahead and smile, it won't be long before someone smiles back!

With every person you meet and greet make your postural muscles switch on, feel elegant and important every time you enter a room whether there are people there or not! You will be amazed at how differently people will think about you.

Try to get up 30 minutes early, throw on your gym kit and go downstairs to your exercise space ready to wake yourself up, get invigorated and make a great start to the day. But some people really aren't morning people, so make sure you train at a time that really suits you, morning, afternoon or evening and mentally prepare yourself for the workout – the difference can be major.

Make your chores part of your exercise plan but speed them up a bit, time yourself while cleaning, dusting, hoovering or mowing the lawn and the next time you do the same jobs, see if you can get them finished a little faster. If you have a small child make a deal about childcare with your partner so you have some time off to exercise. If you can't manage this, increase your heart rate by going for a fast walk with the pushchair. Look at your social calendar and try to get your family involved in a group activity like walking, cycling, badminton, tennis, or go out dancing. Or train with a friend – you'll encourage each other – but make it a regular commitment neither of you will break. Don't be scared to join a class or activity group. You might meet someone who is in the same boat as you; there may be someone looking for a training buddy, and you could be the one to motivate them!

Make sure you get enough sleep to cope with your new lifestyle. If you are not sleeping enough you may find your appetite increases which may cause you to eat sugary foods, and then your metabolism may actually slow down. Go to bed happy. Write down one of the great things that happened to you during the day before you go to sleep, if you do this daily you will soon build up a catalogue of events that will make wonderfully positive reading in the future.

Trouble Shooting

Feeling down … stressed at work … drained and tired … feel like you can't do something? Stop and do the two minute wake-up workout.

- Splash your face with water or take a spritz to work to awaken your senses.
- Focus your breathing, sit (cross-legged if possible) with a strong lengthened back, lift up through your torso, take two slow breaths in and out, swiftly breathe in followed by a more forceful breath out through the nose. Repeat for 2 to 3 minutes.
- When you're sitting, put one hand behind the back and wrap the other over the opposite knee, use the knee to ease yourself around as far as you can rotate through the spine, repeat in the opposite direction.
- Lie on your back, have your legs together, roll the knees in one direction and the head the opposite way to stretch the spine.
- Lie on your back and cuddle the knees into the chest to ease the lower back.
- Turn on to your front and spread the arms slightly wider than the shoulders with the palms facing down, engage your abdominals, push the hands into the floor and lengthen as you lift the upper body away from the floor.
- On all fours, sit back on your heels leaving your arms stretched forwards easing and lengthening through the back.
- Stand up, inhale, exhale, and roll down through the vertebrae keeping the knees soft, working through the back and stretching the legs. Breathe out as you engage navel to spine and begin the journey back up to standing. Repeat 5 times.
- Stand up, spread your arms wide and sway and rotate side to side swinging the arms around the torso releasing the back heel as you turn.

Final Tips — Dos and Don'ts

DO

- eat breakfast, eat sensible portions, cut down on sugar and avoid additives
- exfoliate 2–3 times per week
- massage your body to stimulate the cells – always rub up towards the heart
- reward yourself with a luxurious bath full of oils to help you feel amazing
- drink plenty of water to re-hydrate and flush away toxins
- write a list of all your successes and keep them in view to motivate you
- focus on the body part you are training with 100 per cent attention
- eat plenty of fruit as it has more fibre than grains and contains more antioxidants
- stretch first thing in the morning – smile as you do so for a great start to the day
- make a great CD of all your favourite tunes to work out to
- make landmarks target goals when you are outdoors exercising – this will push you to increase your time and performance and make sure you are keeping on track
- plan your day with realistic targets
- release facial tension by taking deep breaths and chanting the vowels A E I O U
- take time to relax – create the right mood with warm candles and soft music

DON'T

- manage stress by eating or snack when you are bored – do something!
- pile your plate high with food or have second helpings
- say you're too tired to exercise – exercising will give you an energy boost
- slouch
- skip meals
- eat energy bars that may have a high sugar content
- drink excessive alcohol
- treat yourself to a 'bad' food for doing so well
- wear an underwired bra at the gym as it can restrict the blood flow to the breasts
- slip back into your old ways, old habits are the hardest to break, make positive changes that will become new, better habits

You have now adopted a lifestyle that should make you feel 'brand new'. Not only should you know how to look after yourself with food and exercise, but you will know how to manage yourself better. Your inner strength should be greater than ever and you should be walking tall and proud as a reflection of your true self. Ask yourself what values are important to you. Are you, or are you about to be, able to lead and maintain a balanced lifestyle? If not, what could you change to make that happen?

You are in control of your own results. You *can* make this happen. Focus on your positives to achieve more positives, and the rewards will be endless. If you feel you are slipping back, analyse why and be positive in getting rid of the problem.

Treat the cause and the effect will change. Manage the effects and they will remain with you.

Use this book as a simple reference or reminder whenever you feel the need. Call it your pocket personal trainer to assist with your goals. It should lead you to a healthier, happier you, and by now you should have adopted enough key skills to change your life as you choose. Don't look back, keep moving forwards. Enjoy the journey.

Elise
x

GLOSSARY OF MUSCLES

abdominals (abs): stomach muscles which help to give you good posture and a flat stomach

abductors: in the outer thigh – they move the leg outwards

adductors: in the inner thigh – they move the leg inwards

biceps: at the front of the upper arm – they bend the elbow

hamstrings: three large muscles at the back of the leg which bend the knee and straighten the hip

hip flexors: they run from the pelvis and spine to the front of the hip bone and flex the hip

gluteals (glutes): 3 muscles in the bottom – minimus and medius rotate the hip towards the body and move the leg outward; maximus rotates the leg away from the body and moves it inwards

latissimus dorsi: connects the upper arm to the back and draws the arm backwards and towards the body

obliques: bend the body to one side and rotate to the opposite side – these are the muscles that will give you a waist

pectorals: in the front of the chest which pull the shoulders forward and rotate the shoulder joint towards the body

quadriceps (quads): at the front of the thigh which straighten the knee and flex the hip

tibialis anterior: goes from the knee past the ankle and brings the toes up towards your face

trapezius: big muscle in the upper back running from shoulder to shoulder and attaching about mid-spine – upper part lifts the shoulders; lower part draws the shoulder blade down, also rotates the shoulder blade

triceps: muscles in the back of the arm which straighten the elbow